PT Clinical

Notes

A Rehabilitation Pocket Guide

Ellen Hillegass, PT, PhD

809I4900MW

F. A. Davis Company
1915 Arch Street
Philadelphia, PA 19103
www.fadavis.com

Printed in China by Imago

Last digit indicates print number: 10 9 8 7 6 5 4 3 2 1

Senior Acquisitions Editor: Melissa Duffield
Manager of Content Development: George Lang
Manager of Art & Design: Carolyn O'Brien
Developmental Editor: Dean W. DeChambeau
Reviewers: Denise Abrams, PT, DPT, MA; Thomas Bevins, PT, MS; Wendy D. Bircher, PT, EdD; Susan P. Denham, OTR/L, CHT; Weiqing Ge, DPT, PhD; Nathan B. Herz, OTD, MBA, OTR/L, CEAS; You-jou Hung, PT, MS, PhD; Kathleen K. Kelley, EdD, PT, NCS; Kari Christine Inda, PhD, OTR; Michael B. Moore, PhD, ATC; Jackie D. Underwood, PTA, BS

As new scientific information becomes available through basic and clinical research, recommended treatments and drug therapies undergo changes. The author(s) and publisher have done everything possible to make this book accurate, up to date, and in accord with accepted standards at the time of publication. The author(s), editors, and publisher are not responsible for errors or omissions or for consequences from application of the book, and make no warranty, expressed or implied, in regard to the contents of the book. Any practice described in this book should be applied by the reader in accordance with professional standards of care used in regard to the unique circumstances that may apply in each situation. The reader is advised always to check product information (package inserts) for changes and new information regarding dose and contraindications before administering any drug. Caution is especially urged when using new or infrequently ordered drugs.

Place 27/8 x 27/8 **Sticky Notes** here
For a convenient and refillable pad

√ **HIPAA Suportive**
√ **OSHA Compliant**

Waterproof and Reusable
Wipe-Free Pages

Write directly onto any page of *PT Clinical Notes*
with a ballpoint pen. Wipe old entries off
with an alcohol pad and reuse

ASSESS	OUTCOME	ADMIN	MEDSURG	CARDIO	NEURO	MUSCLE	DERMA
H HEALTH	WOMEN	PEDS	LABS	MEDS	WELLNESS	REFS & INDEX	

Look for our other Davis PT Resources

Assessment

The Elements of Patient/Client Management Leading to Optimal Outcomes

DIAGNOSIS

Both the process and the end result of evaluating examination data, which the physical therapist organizes into defined clusters, syndromes, or categories to help determine the prognosis (including the plan of care) and the most appropriate intervention strategies.

PROGNOSIS (INCLUDING PLAN OF CARE)

Determination of the level of optimal improvement that may be attained through intervention and the amount of time required reaching that level. The plan of care specifies the interventions to be used and their timing and frequency.

INTERVENTION

Purposeful and skilled interaction of the physical therapist with patient/client and, if appropriate, with other individuals involved, using various physical therapy procedures and techniques to produce changes in the condition that are consistent with the diagnosis and prognosis. The physical therapist conducts a reexamination to determine changes in patient/client status and to modify or redirect intervention. The decision to reexamine may be based on new clinical findings or on a lack of patient/client progress. The process of reexamination also may identify the need for consultation with or referral to another provider.

OUTCOMES

Results of patient/client management, which include the impact of physical therapy interventions in the following domains: pathology/pathophysiology (disease, disorder, or condition); impairments, functional limitations, and disabilities; risk reduction/prevention; health, wellness, and fitness; societal resources; and patient/client satisfaction.

EXAMINATION

The process of obtaining a history, performing a systems review, and selecting and administering tests and measures to gather data about the patient/client. The initial examination is a comprehensive screening and specific testing process that leads to a diagnostic classification. The examination process also may identify possible problems that require consultation with or referral to another provider.

EVALUATION

A dynamic process in which the physical therapist makes critical judgments based on data gathered during the examination. This process also may identify possible problems that require consultation with or referral to another provider.*

Clinical Problem Solving

1. Identify patient/client's symptoms.
2. Determine symptoms to be addressed.
3. Identify characteristics of relevant symptoms.
4. Develop priority list of problems to be assessed.
5. Identify procedures to examine the symptoms.
6. Perform the examination.
7. Interpret the results of the examination (evaluation).
8. Establish diagnosis.
9. Identify goals and plan of treatment.
10. Provide interventions.
11. Evaluate effect of interventions.
12. Modify treatment program as indicated.

Patient/Client Hx

Chief Complaint & Symptom Hx
- Description of onset of Sx
  - Date of onset
  - Mechanism of injury/disease

*Adapted with permission from American Physical Therapy Association. Guide to Physical Therapist Practice, rev. ed 2. 2003, Alexandria, VA. Fig. 1-4, p. 35.

- Duration of Sx
- Factors that increase Sx
- Factors that decrease Sx
- Associated Sx
  - Patient/client's concerns or needs
  - Prior therapeutic interventions

General Demographics

- Age:
- Sex: __Male__Female
- Race/ethnicity:
  - White
  - African American
  - Hispanic
  - Asian
  - Other
- Primary language:
  - English
  - Spanish
  - French
  - German
  - Japanese
  - Chinese
  - Other
- Education level:
  - K–12; completed grade _____
  - Undergraduate
  - Graduate

Social/Environment Hx

- Family/caregiver resources
- Social supports
- Living environment:
  - Single home
  - Apartment/condominium
  - Senior independent living
  - Assisted living
  - Nursing home
  - Other
    - Use of assistive devices or equipment
- Discharge destination:
  - Same
  - Other

- Social habits:
  - Drinks alcohol__Yes__No   If yes # drinks/wk _____
  - Smokes cigarettes__Yes__No   If yes # cigarettes/day _____
  - If no, former smoker?__Yes__No
  - If yes: # ppd, # years smoked _____
  - Social drug use _____
- Physical fitness: Exercises regularly__Yes__No
- Psychological function:__NL__AB
  - Memory status
  - Depression or anxiety issues

Employment/Occupation
- Currently employed: Yes__No__   Full-time/part-time/other:
  _____ ,
- Occupation: _____
- Retired:__Yes__No
  - If retired, former occupation: _____
- Leisure activities: _____
  _____

Past Medical Hx, Including Surgeries, etc.
- Previous hospitalizations
- Previous surgeries
- Previous medical problems
- Past medical status of problems with:
  - Cardiovascular
  - Endocrine/metabolic
  - Gastrointestinal
  - Genitourinary
  - Gynecological
  - Integumentary
  - Musculoskeletal
  - Neuromuscular
  - Obstetric
  - Psychological
  - Pulmonary

Family Medical Hx
- Fam Hx of cardiovascular disease (angina, heart attack, stroke, CHF, PVD) _____ Age of first Dx _____
- Fam Hx of diabetes _____
- Fam Hx of cancer? Type of cancer? _____
- Other fam Hx _____

4

Functional Status
- Current & prior status in self-care & home management (ADL)
- Work
- Independent
- Requires assistance for self-care or home management
- Dependent in care
- Medication
  - For current condition
  - For other condition

Other Clinical Tests
- Lab & diagnostic
- Other clinical findings

Assessment of Risk Factors

Risk Factors for Falling

Age Changes	Medications
Muscle weakness Decreased balance Impaired proprioception or sensation Delayed muscle response Time/increased reaction time	Antihypertensives Sedative-hypnotics Antidepressants Antipsychotics Diuretics Narcotics Use of more than four medications
Environmental	**Pathological Conditions**
Poor lighting Throw rugs, loose carpet, complex carpet designs Cluster of wires/cords Stairs w/o handrails Bathrooms w/o grab rails Slippery floors Restraints Footwear (slippers) Use of alcohol	Vestibular disorders Orthostatic hypotension (especially before breakfast) Neuropathies Osteoarthritis Osteoporosis Visual or hearing impairment Cardiovascular disease Urinary incontinence CNS disorders (stroke, Parkinson disease, multiple sclerosis)

Continued

Risk Factors for Falling—cont'd

Other	
Elder abuse/assault	Nonambulatory status
Gait changes (decreased stride length or speed)	Postural instability
	Fear of falling

Risk Factors for Heart Disease

CAD Risk Factors	Major = ** Minor = *	Presence = + Absence = − Fam Hx = Fam
Hypertension >140 systolic or >90 diastolic	**	
Smoking (# ppd × # yr)	**	
Elevated cholesterol Total >200, LDL >160 & no CAD *or* LDL >100 w/CAD HDL <40 males, HDL <50 females	**	
Sedentary lifestyle	**	
Fam Hx (1 or more parent <60 yr when dx w/CAD, MI, stroke)	**	
Diabetes	**	
Stress (anger/hostility)	*	
Age (older)	*	
Obesity (M or menopausal F)	*	
Elevated triglycerides >150	*	

Risk Factors for Pulmonary Disease

PD Risk Factors	Presence = + Absence = −
Smoking (ppd × yr smoked)	
Occupational/environmental exposure	

Risk Factors for Pulmonary Disease—cont'd

PD Risk Factors	Presence = + Absence = −
Toxic fume inhalation: chlorine, chemicals, formaldehyde, plant nursery chemicals, etc.	
Dusts: carpentry work, asbestos, coal, silica	
Family Hx of asthma	
Alpha$_1$ antitrypsin deficiency	
AIDS/ARDS	

Risk Factors for Diabetes

- Obesity
- Increased age
- Sedentary lifestyle
- High BP & high cholesterol
- Unhealthy eating habits (high sugar)
- Hx of gestational diabetes
- Family Hx & genetics

Risk Factors for Skin Breakdown

- Amputation
- Surgery
- CHF
- Vascular
- Diabetes
- Altered mentation/coma
- Malnutrition
- Decreased level of activity
- Neuromuscular dysfunction
- Obesity
- Decreased sensation
- Peripheral nerve involvement
- Edema
- Polyneuropathy
- Inflammation

- Prior scar
- Ischemia
- Spinal cord involvement
- Pain

Risk Factors for Deep Vein Thrombosis (DVT)

DVT more likely to occur in people:

- Age >40 yr
- Pregnancy/childbirth: due to hormone changes; risk highest just after childbirth
- Prolonged bedrest (immobility)
- Major injuries or paralysis
- Using contraceptives w/estrogen
- Surgery, especially leg joints or pelvis
- HRT
- Cancer & its treatments
- Other circulation or heart problems
- Long-distance travel: prolonged immobility

Symptoms of DVT
Swelling of leg; warmth & redness of leg; pain, noticeable when standing/walking

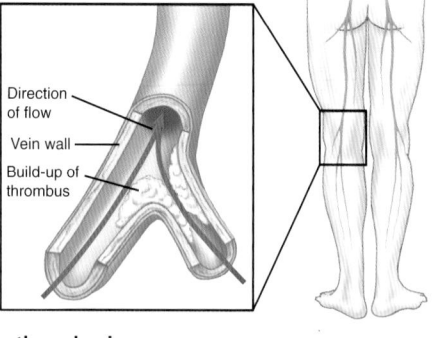

Direction of flow

Vein wall

Build-up of thrombus

Deep vein thrombosis

Wells Clinical Score for DVT

Clinical Parameter Score	Score
Active cancer (treatment ongoing, within 6 mo, or palliative)	+1
Paralysis or recent plaster immobilization of the lower extremities	+1
Recently bedridden for >3 d or major surgery <4 wk	+1
Localized tenderness along the distribution of the deep venous system	+1
Entire leg swelling	+1
Calf swelling >3 cm compared with the asymptomatic leg	+1
Pitting edema (greater in the symptomatic leg)	+1
Previous DVT documented	+1
Collateral superficial veins (nonvaricose)	+1
Alternative diagnosis (as likely or > DVT)	−2
Total of Above Score	
High probability	>3
Moderate probability	1 or 2
Low probability	<0

Adapted from Anand SS, Wells PS, Hunt D, et al. Does this patient have deep vein thrombosis? JAMA. 1998 Apr 8:279(14):1094–9.

Revised Geneva Score to Assess for Risk for DVT

Clinical Pretest Probability of PE

0–3 points is a low, 9% probability of PE

4–10 points is an intermediate, 28% probability of PE

>11 points is a high, 72% probability of PE

Predictor Variable	Score
Age 65 yr or over	1
Previous DVT or PE	3
Surgery or fracture within 1 month	2
Active malignant condition	2
Unilateral lower limb pain	3
Hemoptysis	2
Heart rate 75 to 94 bpm	3
Heart rate 95 or more bpm	5
Pain on deep palpation of lower limb & unilateral edema	4

Pulmonary Embolus

Symptoms of PE
- Shortness of breath (SUDDEN CHANGE)
- Chest pain, w/deep breaths
- Coughing up phlegm w/blood; streaking flecks
- Rapid increase in respiratory rate and/or drop in SpO₂

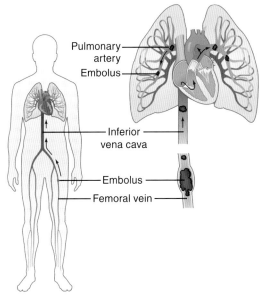

Pulmonary embolism

Systems Review

Cardiovascular/Pulmonary	NL	ABN
Resting BP (<140/90)		
Resting HR (<100 bpm)		
Resting RR (<16 breaths/min)		
Edema		
BMI <25		
• Bilateral		
• Unilateral		

Integumentary	NL	ABN
Pliability (texture)		
Presence of scar formation		
Skin color		
Skin integrity		

Musculoskeletal: ROM & Strength	NL	ABN
Gross ROM		
• UE		
• LE		
Gross strength		
• UE		
• LE		
Symmetry		
Height		
Wt		
BMI		

Systems Review—cont'd		
Neuromuscular	**NL**	**ABN**
Gross coordinated movements		
Balance		
• Sitting		
• Standing		
Gait		
Locomotion		
Transfers		
Transitions		
Motor function/motor control		
Gastrointestinal/Genitourinary	**NL**	**ABN**
Heartburn, diarrhea, vomiting, abdominal pain		
Menstrual problems, pregnancy		
Swallowing problems		
Bladder problems: continence? urgency?		
Bowel problems: continence?		
Communication/Affect/Cognition/Language/Learning Style	**NL**	**ABN**
Ability to make needs known		
Consciousness		
Expected emotional/behavioral responses		
Learning preferences/education needs/barriers		
Orientation (person, place, time)		
General	**NL**	**ABN**
Unexplained wt loss or gain		
Fever, chills, fatigue		

Standing Balance Test

Pt should maintain position w/o moving or swaying.

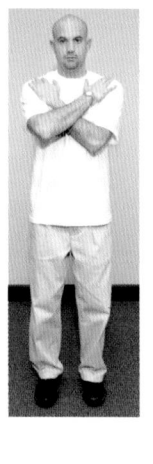

Body Mass Index Table

	Normal						Overweight					Obese										Extreme obesity		
BMI	19	20	21	22	23	24	25	26	27	28	29	30	31	32	33	34	35	36	37	38	39	40	41	42
Height (inches)												**Body Weight (pounds)**												
58	91	96	100	105	110	115	119	124	129	134	138	143	148	153	158	162	167	172	177	181	186	191	196	201
59	94	99	104	109	114	119	124	128	133	138	143	148	153	158	163	168	173	178	183	188	193	198	203	208
60	97	102	107	112	118	123	128	133	138	143	148	153	158	163	168	174	179	184	189	194	199	204	209	215
61	100	106	111	116	122	127	132	137	143	148	153	158	164	169	174	180	185	190	195	201	206	211	217	222
62	104	109	115	120	126	131	136	142	147	153	158	164	169	175	180	186	191	196	202	207	213	218	224	229
63	107	113	118	124	130	135	141	146	152	158	163	169	175	180	186	191	197	203	208	214	220	225	231	237
64	110	116	122	128	134	140	145	151	157	163	169	174	180	186	192	197	204	209	215	221	227	232	238	244
65	114	120	126	132	138	144	150	156	162	168	174	180	186	192	198	204	210	216	222	228	234	240	246	252
66	118	124	130	136	142	148	155	161	167	173	179	186	192	198	204	210	216	223	229	235	241	247	253	260
67	121	127	134	140	146	153	159	166	172	178	185	191	198	204	211	217	223	230	236	242	249	255	261	268
68	125	131	138	144	151	158	164	171	177	184	190	197	203	210	216	223	230	236	243	249	256	262	269	276
69	128	135	142	149	155	162	169	176	182	189	196	203	209	216	223	230	236	243	250	257	263	270	277	284
70	132	139	146	153	160	167	174	181	188	195	202	209	216	222	229	236	243	250	257	264	271	278	285	292
71	136	143	150	157	165	172	179	186	193	200	208	215	222	229	236	243	250	257	265	272	279	286	293	301
72	140	147	154	162	169	177	184	191	199	206	213	221	228	235	242	250	258	265	272	279	287	294	302	309
73	144	151	159	166	174	182	189	197	204	212	219	227	235	242	250	257	265	272	280	288	295	302	310	318
74	148	155	163	171	179	186	194	202	210	218	225	233	241	249	256	264	272	280	287	295	303	311	319	326
75	152	160	168	176	184	192	200	208	216	224	232	240	248	256	264	272	279	287	295	303	311	319	327	335
76	156	164	172	180	189	197	205	213	221	230	238	246	254	263	271	279	287	295	304	312	320	328	336	344

BMI = body mass (kg)/height (m)
Adapted from Clinical Guidelines on the Identification, Evaluation, and Treatment of Overweight and Obesity in Adults: The Evidence Report, NIH publication 98–4083, September 1998.

Questions Designed to Engage the Patient/ Client in the Treatment Planning Process

1. What are your concerns?
2. What is your greatest concern?
3. What would you like to see happen? What would make you feel that you are making progress in dealing with your chief concern?
5. What are your goals?
6. What is your specific goal?

Ozer, 2000.

Tests & Measures: Areas in Systems Areas in Systems Review Requiring Further Assessment

Cardiovascular & Pulmonary

- Aerobic capacity/endurance tests
  - Functional capacity during ADL
    - Standardized exercise testing protocols
      - 6-minute walk test
- Cardiovascular S&S in response to increased O_2 demand w/exercise or activity
  - HR, rhythm, heart sounds
  - BP, arterial pressures, pulses, blood flow (w/Doppler)
  - Perceived exertion w/activities
  - Angina, claudication assessments
    - Anthropometric characteristics
- Pulmonary S&S in response to increased O_2 demand w/activity or exercise
  - Dyspnea
  - SpO_2
  - Ventilatory pattern
  - Cyanosis, gas exchange, gas analysis
- Physiological responses to position change, including autonomic responses, central, & peripheral pressures
- Pulmonary signs of ventilatory function
  - Airway protection
  - Breath & voice sounds
  - Respiratory rate, rhythm, & pattern

- Ventilatory flow, forces, & volumes
- Airway clearance assessment

Neuromuscular

- Neuromotor development & sensory integration
  - Arousal, attention, & cognition
  - Cranial & peripheral nerve integrity
  - Response to neural provocation
  - Reflex integrity
  - Response to stimuli (auditory, gustatory, olfactory, pharyngeal, vestibular, & visual)
  - Sensory distribution of cranial & peripheral nerves
  - Discrimination tests
  - Tactile tests
  - Coarse vs. light touch
  - Cold vs. heat tests
  - Pressure/vibration tests
  - Dexterity, coordination, & agility tests
  - Pain
  - Electroneuromyography
- Initiation, modification, & control of movement patterns
  - Developmental scales
  - Movement assessment batteries
  - Postural challenge tests

Musculoskeletal Assessment

- Dynamometry
- Specific muscle tests
  - Hand function: fine vs. gross motor, finger dexterity
  - Joint integrity & mobility
  - Apprehension, compression, & distraction
  - Drawer, glide, impingement, shear, & valgus/varus stress tests
  - Joint play movements
  - Muscle strength, power, & endurance tests
  - Muscle tension (palpation)
  - Muscle length, soft-tissue extensibility, & flexibility tests
  - Posture evaluation
  - Ergonomics & body mechanics
  - Range of motion & muscle length
- Thoracic outlet tests

- vertebral artery compression
- Orthotic, protective, & supportive devices
- Prosthetic requirements
- Environmental, home, & work barriers
- Assistive & adaptive devices
- Self-care & home management
- Work, community, & leisure integration

Integumentary

- Activities, positions, & postures that produce or relieve trauma
- Assessment of devices/equipment that produce or relieve trauma to skin
- Skin characteristics
  - Blistering
  - Mobility of skin
  - Dermatitis
  - Nail growth
  - Hair growth
  - Temperature, texture, turgor

Functional Tests		
	Test	**Assistance**
Bed mobility	Rolling side to side	
	Scooting up & down in bed	
Transfers	Supine ↔ Sidelying ↔ Sit	
	Sit ↔ Stand	
	Stand pivot sit	
	Wheelchair ↔ Toilet	
	Wheelchair ↔ Tub	
Balance	Sitting	
	Standing	
	Dynamic	
Ambulation	w/Assistive device	
	w/o Assistive device	

Functional Assessment & Impairment Terminology Definitions

Independent	Pt able to consistently perform skill safely w/no one present & no cuing
Supervision	Pt requires one person w/in arm's reach as precaution; ↓ probability of requiring assistance
Close guarding	Person positioned to assist w/hands raised but not touching pt; fair probability of requiring assistance
Minimum assist	Pt completes **majority** of activity w/o assist
Moderate assist	Pt completes **part** of activity w/o assist
Maximum assist	Pt unable to assist in any part of activity

Balance Definitions: Sitting or Standing

NL	Maintains position w/maximal disturbance
Good	Maintains position w/moderate disturbance
Fair	Maintains position unsupported: short period
Poor	Attempts to assist: requires assist to maintain
None	Unable to assist in maintaining position

20

Pain Assessment

Wong-Baker FACES® Pain Rating Scale

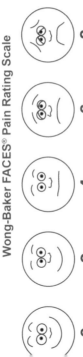

0	2	4	6	8	10
No Hurt	Hurts Little Bit	Hurts Little More	Hurts Even More	Hurts Whole Lot	Hurts Worst

©1983 Wong-Baker FACES® Foundation. Visit us at www.wongbakerFACES.org.
Used with permission. Originally published in Whaley & Wong's Nursing Care of Infants and Children. ©Elsevier Inc.

From Meyers, E. R. Notes: Nurse's Clinical Pocket Guide. Philadelphia, F.A. Davis Co., 2003, p. 29.

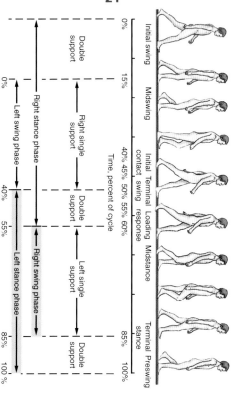

Gait

Initial swing | Midswing | Initial Terminal Loading Midstance | Terminal Preswing
contact swing response | stance

Time, percent of cycle

0% | 15% | 40% 45% 50% 55% 60% | 40% 55% | 85% 100%

Double support

Right single support

Left swing phase

Double support

Left single support

Right swing phase

Double support

Left stance phase

Right stance phase

Adapted from Inman VT, Ralston HJ, Todd F: Human Walking, Baltimore, 1981, Williams & Wilkins. Figure 32-1 Phases of the gait cycle. In Magee DJ: Orthopedic Physical Assessment, ed 4, St. Louis, 2002, WB Saunders.

Communication w/Nonverbal Patient/Client

YES   NO

THANK YOU

I NEED

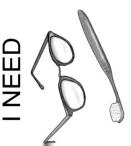

PLEASE TURN   ON   OFF

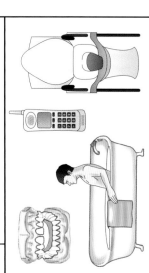

Special Considerations w/All Populations: Alerts/Indicators

Effects of Bedrest

↓ VO₂ max	Muscle atrophy
↓ Plasma volume	↓ Muscle tone
↓ Red blood cell mass	↓ Muscle endurance
↓ Stroke volume	Bone demineralization
↓ Maximal exercise cardiac output	↓ Insulin sensitivity
↓ Oxidative capacity of muscle	↓ Carbohydrate tolerance
↓ Orthostatic tolerance	↑ Serum lipids
↓ Vasomotor function	Altered immune system function
↓ Heat tolerance	↑ Susceptibility to infection, DVT, sleep disturbance
↓ Nitrogen balance in skeletal muscle	

Effects of Aging on Body Functions

↓ Peak VO₂ (aerobic capacity)	↓ 20%–30% by age 80 yr
↓ Cardiac index	↓ 20%–30% by age 80 yr
↓ Max breathing capacity	↓ 40%
↓ Liver & kidney function	↓ 40%–50%
↓ Bone mass	↓ 15% in men, 30% in women
↓ Muscle strength	↓ 20%–30%
↓ Joint flexibility	↓ 20%–30%
↓ Endocrine function	↓ 40%
↓ # Spinal cord axons	↓ 37%
↓ Nerve conduction velocity	↓ 10%–15%

Signs & Symptoms of Physical Abuse

The Elderly
- Bruises, black eyes, welts, lacerations, & rope marks
- Bone fractures, broken bones, & skull fractures
- Open wounds, cuts, punctures, untreated injuries in various stages of healing
- Sprains, dislocations, & internal injuries/bleeding

punishment, & signs of being restrained
- Laboratory findings of medication overdose or underutilization of prescribed drugs
- An elder's report of being hit, slapped, kicked, or mistreated
- An elder's sudden change in behavior
- The caregiver's refusal to allow visitors to see an elder alone

Children & Adolescents
- Unexplained burns, cuts, bruises, or welts in the shape of an object
- Fear of adults
- Bite marks
- Drug or alcohol abuse
- Antisocial behavior
- Self-destructive or suicidal behavior
- Problems in school
- Depression or poor self-image

Some Signs of Emotional Abuse
- Apathy
- Overcompliance or excessive aggression
- Depression
- Hostility
- Fear of a particular person or fam member
- Lack of concentration
- Eating disorders
- Withdrawal, secretiveness, or depression
- Inappropriate interest in or knowledge of sexual acts
- Suicidal behavior
- Seductiveness
- Eating disorders
- Self-injury
- Substance abuse
- Avoidance of things related to sexuality or rejection of own genitals or body
- Running away
- Nightmares & bedwetting
- Inhibited behavior
- Drastic changes in appetite
- Disturbed play
- Aggression

Nutritional Needs Assessment

% Ideal body wt. _____ BMI_____
Wt. change: Mild _____ Moderate _____ Severe _____
Available lab reports: Albumin _____ Cholesterol: _____
Glucose _____
Possible drug/nutrient reactions: _____
Comments/assessment _____

Indicators of Nutritional Problems	Yes	No
Significant wt change (+/– 10 lb or > in past year)		
Intermittent or continuous use of steroids		
>30% BMI		
Changes in eating habits recently		
Follows dietary restrictions		
Food allergies		
Problems with:		
• Dental		
• Chewing		
• Swallowing		
• Digestion		
• Constipation/diarrhea		
Inadequate intake of fluids (<8 cups or 64 oz/d)		
Low albumin/prealbumin		

Red Flags for Potential Feeding Difficulties	
Slow feeding progression	Tube feeding beyond 2 mo
Respiratory difficulties	Persistent reflexes
Spits out food	Jaw moves excessively
Oral touch sensitive	ABN muscle tone
Anoxic events	Color change w/feeding
Coughs frequently	Poor transition to solids
Hypersensitive gag	

Continued

Nutritional Needs Assessment—cont'd

Red Flags for Swallowing Difficulties

Hx of respiratory difficulties	Stridor
Pneumonias	Color changes
Muscle tone abnormalities	Coughing during or after feeding
Traumatic brain injury	Poor handling of secretions
Ventilator dependence	Slow growth pattern
Apnea	

PT Education Needs Assessment Checklist

- ☐ Understanding of disease
- ☐ Knowledge of medications: indications & side effects
- ☐ Activity limitations
- ☐ S&S to anticipate
- ☐ Action to take w/S&S
- ☐ Knowledge of when to call doctor/ER
- ☐ Readiness to learn
- ☐ Use of caregivers
- ☐ Self-management of disease

Additional PT Resources

- ☐ Dietitian
- ☐ Psychologist/behav specialist
- ☐ Case mgr/social worker
- ☐ Other specialist

Hospital/Home

Adaptive Equipment Chart

Equipment	Have	Need	Special Considerations
Hospital bed			
Wheelchair			
• Manual			
• Electric			
Mobility			
• Cane: straight			
• 4-pronged			
• Walker			
• Pickup			
• 2 wheels			
• 4 wheels			
Raised toilet seat			
Shower/bath stool			
Electric bed			
Grab bars in bathroom			
Other			

Adaptive Equipment & Environment Dimensions

Wheelchair dimensions	
Overall height	36–37 in
Seat depth	16–17 in
Footrest support	16–22 in
Armrest height	5–12 in
Seat height from floor	19.5–20.5 in
Seat & back width	14–22 in

Wheelchair clearance for door	36 in min
Turning space for wheelchair	60–78 in min
Closet: hanging or shelf heights	48 in max
Drinking fountains spout height	36 in max
Bathroom stall	60 × 96 in
Bathtubs: clear space out of tub	60 × 30 in

Wheelchair Measurement

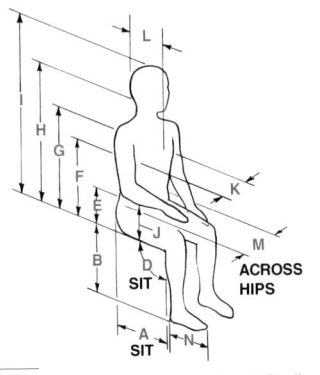

From Hillegass, E.A. Sadowsky, H.S. Essentials of Cardiopulmonary Physical Therapy, ed. 2. WB Saunders, Philadelphia, 2001.

Discharge: Expected

Assessment of Planned Destination: Acute Rehab/Skilled Care/Home

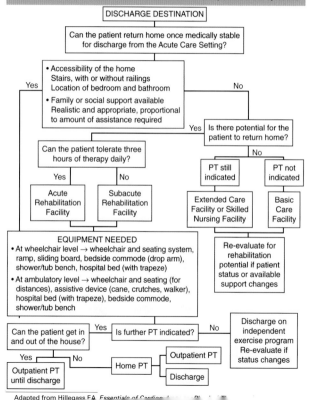

DISCHARGE DESTINATION

Can the patient return home once medically stable for discharge from the Acute Care Setting?

- Accessibility of the home
  Stairs, with or without railings
  Location of bedroom and bathroom
- Family or social support available
  Realistic and appropriate, proportional
  to amount of assistance required

Yes

No

Is there potential for the patient to return home?

Yes

No

Can the patient tolerate three hours of therapy daily?

Yes → Acute Rehabilitation Facility

No → Subacute Rehabilitation Facility

PT still indicated

PT not indicated

Extended Care Facility or Skilled Nursing Facility

Basic Care Facility

Re-evaluate for rehabilitation potential if patient status or available support changes

EQUIPMENT NEEDED
- At wheelchair level → wheelchair and seating system, ramp, sliding board, bedside commode (drop arm), shower/tub bench, hospital bed (with trapeze)
- At ambulatory level → wheelchair and seating (for distances), assistive device (cane, crutches, walker), hospital bed (with trapeze), bedside commode, shower/tub bench

Can the patient get in and out of the house?

Yes → Is further PT indicated?

No → Discharge on independent exercise program Re-evaluate if status changes

Yes / No

Home PT → Outpatient PT / Discharge

Outpatient PT until discharge

Adapted from Hillegass EA. Essentials of Cardiopulmonary Physical Therapy

Procedural Interventions

Based on outcomes one wishes to achieve, the following are options for procedures or interventions in PT practice:

- ADL training
- Aerobic capacity/endurance conditioning or reconditioning
- Airway clearance techniques
- Balance, coordination, & agility training
- Body mechanics & postural stabilization
- Breathing strategies
- Coordination, communication, & documentation
- Devices & equipment use & training
- Electrotherapeutic modalities
- Flexibility exercise
- Functional training programs in self-care, home management, work community, & leisure
- Gait & locomotion training
- Injury prevention or reduction
- Integumentary repair & protection techniques
- Manual therapy techniques & mobilization/manipulation
- Neuromotor development training
- Pt/client-related instruction
- Physical agents & mechanical modalities
- Positioning
- Prescription, application, & fabrication of devices & equipment
- Relaxation training
- Strength, power, & endurance training for skeletal & ventilatory muscles

APTA, 2001.

Anticipated or Expected Outcomes

- Ability to perform physical actions/tasks/activities improved
- Ability to perform, assume, or resume required self-care, home management, work, etc. ↑
- Aerobic capacity improved
- Airway clearance improved
- Atelectasis ↓

- ■ Balance improved
- ■ Cough improved
- ■ Edema, lymphedema, or effusion ↓
- ■ Endurance ↑
- ■ Energy expenditure per unit of work ↓
- ■ Exercise tolerance improved
- ■ Fitness improved
- ■ Gait, locomotion, & balance improved
- ■ Health status improved
- ■ Integumentary integrity improved
- ■ Joint integrity & mobility improved
- ■ Joint swelling, inflammation, or restriction reduced
  - ■ Level of supervision required for task performance ↓
  - ■ Motor function (motor control & motor learning) improved
  - ■ Muscle performance (strength, power, & endurance) ↑
  - ■ Optimal joint alignment achieved
  - ■ Optimal loading on a body part achieved
  - ■ Pain decreased
  - ■ Performance of ADLs with or w/o assistive devices ↑
  - ■ Physical function improved
  - ■ Physiological response to ↑ O_2 demand improved
  - ■ Postural control improved
  - ■ Pre- & postoperative complications ↓
  - ■ Quality & quantity of movement of body segments improved
  - ■ ROM improved
  - ■ Relaxation ↑
  - ■ Risk of secondary impairment ↓
  - ■ Risk factors for disease ↓
  - ■ Self-mgmt of Sx improved
  - ■ Sensory awareness ↑
  - ■ Soft tissue swelling, inflammation, or restriction ↓
  - ■ Tissue perfusion & oxygenation enhanced
  - ■ Tolerance of positions & activities ↑
  - ■ Use of physical therapy services optimized
  - ■ Use & cost of health-care services ↓
  - ■ Weight-bearing status improved
  - ■ Work of breathing ↓

APTA, 2001.

Functional Assessment Outcome Tools

Test	Description
Barthel Index	Measures functional independence in ADLs
Borg Rating of Perceived Exertion	Perceived effort w/activity (6–20 scale or 0–10 scale)
Box and Block Test	Gross dexterity w/grasp & release/unilateral assessment
Canadian Occupational Performance Measure	Pt/client's assessment of performance in self-care over time
Chair Rise Tests	Assesses lower extremity functional strength 1. Assess pt/client's ability to rise from chair one time, OR 2. Assess pt/client's ability to rise from chair 5 times, measuring the amount of time it takes (normative values exist) 3. Count number of times pt/client can rise from & return to chair in 30 sec
Clinical Outcome Variable Scale	Assessment of physical mobility
Disabilities of the Arm, Shoulder, & Hand	UE disability quantified: physical, social, & Sx measures
Functional Assessment System of Lower Extremity Dysfunction	LE function in arthritic pt/client (20 variables, 5-point scale)
Functional Independence Measure	Functional independence assessed in 23 items
Functional Reach Test	Assesses dynamic balance while reaching
Gait Speed Measurement	Using either 6 m or 20 m measured distance, measure time pt/client walks either 4 m or 10 m: compares to individual's function

Functional Assessment Outcome Tools—cont'd

Test	Description
Glittre ADL test	Functional test carrying backpack (for those who carry O_2), walking, 2-stair climb, UE reaching and return
Grocery Shelving Test	UE functional test: placing cans on shelf 15 cm above shoulder level
Katz ADL index	Degree of dependence (8-point scale): mostly in elderly, also used in children
Kenny Self-Care Evaluation	Assessment of ADLs
Klein-Bell ADL Scale	Assessment of ADLs of adults w/disability (170 items)
Level of Rehabilitation Scale	Assessment of independence in ADLs, mobility, & communication
Lower Extremity Activity Profile	LE function (self-care & mobility: 23 items)
Lower Extremity Functional Scale	LE function in pts/clients w/musculoskeletal disorders (20 items)
Older Americans Resources & Services Scale–Instrumental Activities of Daily Living	Functional ability & needs for home services in older adults
Patient Evaluation Conference System	Changes in function in pts/clients in rehabilitation (79 items)
Patient Specific Functional Scale	Self Report: patient reports 5 activities he/she has difficulty performing and rates on scale 1–10 for each
PULSES Profile	Function in chronically ill institutionalized persons
Rivermead Mobility Index	Mobility in pts/clients w/neurological conditions

Continued

Test	Description
Rhomberg Balance Tests	Balance evaluations/screens including Rhomberg and Modified: (30-sec balance screen)
Seattle Angina Questionnaire	Assess function in pts/clients w/angina Sx
Self-Paced Walking Test	Estimate max O_2 uptake following walk of 128 m at 3 paces
Short Physical Performance Battery (SPPB)	Assessment of function by looking at chair rise time (lower extremity strength), modified Rhomberg (balance), & gait speed (correlates w/function)
Timed Walk Tests (3-, 6-, 12-min)	Functional performance during ambulation: originally tested in chronic lung disease pts/clients
Timed Stands Test	Lower extremity strength in pts/clients w/arthritis
Timed "Up and Go" Test	Mobility of frail elderly: timed rise from chair, walk for 3 m, return to sit
Upper Extremity Functional Scale	UE function in the workplace
Visual Analogue Scale for Dyspnea	Pt/client's perceptions of dyspnea; used w/activities

Disease Management Outcomes

Cardiac Rehabilitation Outcomes

Outcome Classification	Options	
Behavioral Outcomes	Diet: compliance w/diet, wt mgmt Exercise: compliance w/exercise program Smoking cessation	Stress reduction Able to recognize S&S Medical mgmt Sexual function
Clinical Outcomes	Weight BMI BP Lipids Functional capacity Blood nicotine levels O₂ saturation	Symptom mgmt Psychosocial: return to vocation/leisure, psych status Medical utilization, hospitalizations, meds, physician, or ER visits
Health Outcomes	Morbidity Mortality QOL	Future events: MI, CABG, angioplasty, new angina, serious arrhythmias
Service	Pt/client satisfaction	

Pulmonary Rehabilitation Outcomes

Domains	Outcome Measures	
Behavior	Smoking cessation Breathing retraining Coping strategies Bronchial hygiene Medication adherence	Supplemental O₂ use Pacing techniques Energy conservation Sexual function Adherence to diet
Clinical	Fatigue Depression/anxiety Physical performance measures	Exercise tolerance/exercise performance on walk test Exertional dyspnea Dyspnea w/specific ADLs
Health	Mortality Health-related QOL Morbidity: no rehospitalizations, time between physician visits for illness, health-care utilization, lack of ER visits	
Service	Pt/client satisfaction	

Functional Independence Measure (FIM)

Assesses Cognitive & Physical Disability
Seven Levels of Scoring for Each Measure

7. Complete independence: Fully independent (timely, safely)
6. Modified independence: Requiring the use of a device but no physical help
5. Supervision: Requiring only standby assistance or verbal prompting or help w/setup
4. Minimal assistance: Requiring incidental hands-on help only (subject performs 75% or more of the task)
3. Moderate assistance: Subject still performs 50%–74% of the task
2. Maximal assistance: Subject provides <50% of the effort (25%–49%)
1. Total assistance: Subject contributes <25% of the effort or is unable to do the task

Measures

Self-Care

1. Eating	5. Dressing lower body
2. Grooming	6. Toileting
3. Bathing/showering	7. Swallowing
4. Dressing upper body	

Sphincters

1. Bladder management
2. Bowel management

Mobility

1. Transfers: bed/chair/wheelchair	5. Locomotion: walking/wheelchair
2. Transfers: toilet	6. Locomotion: stairs
3. Transfers: bathtub/shower	7. Community mobility
4. Transfers: car	

Communication

1. Expression	4. Writing
2. Comprehension	5. Speech intelligibility
3. Reading	

Psychosocial

1. Social interaction	3. Adjustment to limitations
2. Emotional status	4. Use of leisure time (replaces employability in original version)

Functional Independence Measure (FIM)—cont'd

Cognition

1. Problem solving 2. Memory 3. Orientation	4. Concentration (replaces attention in original version) 5. Safety awareness (replaces safety judgment in original version)

Scoring Principles

Function is assessed on the basis of direct observation. The subject is scored on what he/she actually does on a day-to-day basis, not on what he/she could do.

Admission scoring is done within 10 days of admission.

Discharge scoring is done during the last week before discharge.

Scoring is done by a multidisciplinary team member.

Do not leave any score blank. Score 1 if the subject does not perform the activity at all, or if no information is available. If function is variable, use the lower score. The official FIM scale requires certification.

Reproduced with the permission of L Turner-Stokes from Turner-Stokes L, Nyein K, Turner-Stokes T et al. The UK FIM+FAM: development and evaluation. Clin Rehabil. 1999; 13: 277–87.

Health Status/Quality of Life Outcome Tools

Test	Description
Arthritis Impact Measurement Scales	Quantifies health status of RA over physical, social, & mental domains
Chronic Respiratory Disease Questionnaire	QOL in pts/clients w/chronic lung disease
EuroQOL-5D (European Quality of Life Scale)	Health-care QOL
Ferrans-Powers QOL tools	Health-related quality of life tools for all diseases
Health Utilities Index	Health-related QOL
Kansas City Cardiomyopathy QOL	QOL for pts/clients w/congestive heart failure behavioral outcomes

Continued

Health Status/Quality of Life Outcome Tools—cont'd

Test	Description
Living With Heart Failure Questionnaire	QOL in pts/clients w/congestive heart failure
Nottingham Health Profile	Health status w/musculoskeletal disorders (38 items)
St. George's Respiratory Questionnaire	Health-related QOL in pts/clients w/chronic lung disease
Short Form Health Survey (SF-36)	Perceived health status; nondisease-specific (36 items)
12-Item Short Form Health Survey	Shorter version of SF-36
Sickness Inventory Profile	Perceived health status in nondisease-specific populations

Musculoskeletal-Specific Outcome Tools

	Test	Description
Spine/Low Back-Specific	Dual inclinometer method of measuring spinal mobility	Spinal mobility
	Inclinometer method (single) of measuring spinal mobility	Spinal mobility
	Modified Schober method for measuring spinal mobility	Spinal mobility
	Numeric Pain Rating Scale	Pain intensity in pts/clients w/muscular disorders
	Oswestry Low Back Pain Disability Questionnaire	Perceived disability due to low back pain
	Roland & Morris Disability Questionnaire	Disability index for pts/clients w/low back pain
	Sorensen Test for Endurance of Back Muscles	Back muscle function (in prone position)
	Visual Analogue Scale for Pain	Pt/client's perceptions of pain; used w/activities

Musculoskeletal-Specific Outcome Tools—cont'd

UE-Specific	Box and Block Test	Gross dexterity w/grasp & release/ unilateral assessment
	Disabilities of the arm, shoulder, & hand	UE disability quantified: physical, social, & Sx measures
	Upper Extremity Functional Scale	UE function in the workplace
	Wolf Motor Function Test	Assesses speed of movement in 15 UE movements post traumatic brain injury & CVA
LE-specific	Functional Assessment System of Lower Extremity Dysfunction	LE function in arthritic pts/clients (20 variables, 5-point scale)
	Lower Extremity Activity Profile	LE function (self-care & mobility: 23 items)
	Lower Extremity Functional Scale	LE function in pts/clients w/muscular disorders (20 items)
	Timed Stands Test	LE strength in pts/clients w/arthritis

Pediatric-Specific Outcome Tools

Alberta Infant Motor Scale	Assesses delays in development of motor performance: 58 items
Bayley Scales of Infant Development	Functional development from 1–42 mo
Bruininks-Oseretsky Test of Motor Proficiency	Developmental motor functioning for ages 4.5–14.5 yr (46 items)
Gross Motor Function Measure	Gross motor function in children w/cerebral palsy & Down syndrome compared w/5-yr-old child
Gross Motor Performance Measure	Quality of movement in children w/cerebral palsy (20 items)
Peabody Developmental Motor Scale, 2nd ed.	Gross & fine motor skills in children from birth to 6 yr

Continued

Pediatric-Specific Outcome Tools—cont'd

Pediatric Evaluation of Disability Inventory	Mobility, self-care, & social function 6 mo–7 yr
WeeFIM (Functional Independence for Children)	Change in disability in children over time

Stroke-Specific Outcome Tools

Test	Items Examined
Action Research Arm Test	UE function after a stroke: 4 subscales
Canadian Neurological Scale	Post acute CVA neuro-status: mental status, motor function, & response
Chedoke-McMaster Stroke Assessment	Impairments & disability post CVA
Emory Functional Ambulation Profile	Assessment of ambulation capability post CVA
Frenchay Arm Test	Arm function recovery post CVA
Fugi-Meyer Assessment of Sensorimotor Recovery After Stroke	Recovery post CVA
Motor Assessment Scale	Motor recovery post CVA
Stroke-Adapted Sickness Impact Profile	QOL post CVA
Stroke Impact Scale	Functional assessment post CVA
Wolf Motor Function Test	Assesses speed of movement in 15 UE movements post traumatic brain injury & CVA

Other Outcome Tools

Balance	Activity-Specific Balance Confidence Scale	Determine confidence in not losing balance: 16-item scale
	Berg Balance Scale	Balance/maintenance of posture w/14 challenges
	Functional Reach Test	Balance
Depression	Beck Depression Inventory	Depression and/or anxiety Sx & function
	Center for Epidemiologic Depression Scales CES-D	
	Hospital Anxiety Depression Study (HADS)	
Diet Assessment	Diet Habit Survey	Saturated fat, salt, & complex carbohydrate intake
	MEDFICTS (meat, eggs, dairy, fried foods, baked goods, convenience foods, table fats, snacks)	Dietary fat intake
Pain Assessment	Numeric Pain Rating Scale	Pain intensity in pts/clients w/musculoskeletal disorders
	Visual Analogue Scale for Pain	Pt/client's perceptions of pain; used w/activities

Modified from Rothstein, Roy, & Wolf: The Rehabilitation Specialist's Handbook, Table 8–3, FA Davis, 2005.

Reimbursement Coding

Therapists often use the following American Medical Association Current Procedural Terminology (CPT) codes when charging for services. Providers of rehabilitation therapy services must refer to their Local Medicare Review Policy (LMRP) and private insurance carriers regarding payment for services when using these codes. Therapists must also check whether these codes can be used for the specific ICD-9 diagnostic code(s) assigned to each patient/client when referred to therapy. See AMA *Guide to CPT Coding* for information on CPT coding and descriptions. To identify LMRPs for therapy services: cms.hhs.gov/mcd/search.asp

Common CPT Codes Used in Therapy

(*are timed codes)

Code	Service
93797	Cardiac rehab (incident to physician) without continuous ECG monitoring
93798	Cardiac rehab (incident to physician) *with* continuous ECG monitoring
94620	Simple exercise test (with or without oxygen monitoring)
94640	Demonstration and/or evaluation of pt/client utilization of an aerosol generator, nebulizer, metered dose inhaler, or IPPB device
94664	*Demonstration and/or evaluation* of pt/client utilization of an aerosol generator, nebulizer, metered dose inhaler, or IPPB device
94667	Manipulation of chest wall, such as cupping, percussing, and vibration to facilitate lung function; *initial demonstration and/or evaluation*
94668	Manipulation of chest wall, such as cupping, percussing, and vibration to facilitate lung function; *subsequent*

Common CPT Codes Used in Therapy—cont'd

Code	Service
97001	Physical therapy evaluation
97002	Physical therapy reevaluation
97005	Occupational therapy evaluation
97010	Hot or cold packs
97012	Traction, mechanical
97014	Electrical stimulation (unattended)
97016	Vasopneumatic services
97018	Paraffin bath
97020	Microwave
97022	Whirlpool
97024	Diathermy
97026	Infrared
97028	Ultraviolet
97032*	Electrical stimulation (manual), 15 min
97033*	Iontophoresis
97034*	Contrast baths, 15 min
97035*	Ultrasound, 15 min
97036*	Hubbard tank, 15 min
97039	Unlisted modality
97110*	Therapeutic exercise, 15 min
97112*	Neuromuscular reeducation, 15 min
97113*	Aquatic therapy with therapeutic exercise, 15 min
97116*	Gait training, 15 min
97124*	Massage, 15 min
97139	Unlisted physical medicine procedure
97140*	Manual therapy techniques, 15 min
97150	Therapeutic procedures, group

Continued

Common CPT Codes Used in Therapy—cont'd

Code	Service
97504*	Orthotics fitting and training, 15 min
97520*	Prosthetics training, 15 min
97530*	Therapeutic activities, 15 min
97532*	Development of cognitive skills, one-on-one, each 15 min
97533*	Sensory integrative techniques, one-on-one, each 15 min
97535*	Self-care and home management, 15 min
97537*	Community/work reintegration, 15 min
97542*	Wheelchair management/propulsion training, 15 min
97545	Work hardening/conditioning, initial 2 h
97546	Work hardening/conditioning, each additional h
97597	Removal of devitalized tissue from wound, selective débridement w/o anesthesia, less than or equal to 20 sq cm
97598	Débridement of total wound surface area >20 sq cm
97602	Non-selective débridement
97605	Negative pressure wound therapy; total wound surface area < or equal to 50 sq cm
97606	Negative pressure wound therapy, total wound surface area >50 sq cm
97703*	Checkout for orthotic/prosthetic use, estab pt/client, each 15 min
97750*	Physical performance test or measurement, each 15 min (report required to accompany claim)
97755	Assistive technology assessment
G0422	Intensive cardiac rehab services w/exercise
G0423	Intensive cardiac rehab services w/o exercise
G0424	Pulmonary rehab services* (only used with COPD diagnosis)

NOTE: Only *one* evaluation code can be billed during each daily session.

Time Increments for Billing Purposes

Time (min)	0–<8	>7–<23	>22–<38	>37–<53	>52–<68
Billable time (units)	0	1	2	3	4

Modifiers Used

-22	Unusual procedural services
-52	Reduced services
-59	Distinct procedural service
-76	Repeat procedure by same physician
-32	Mandated services (e.g., workers compensation requires functional capacity evaluation)
-99	Multiple modifiers
-GA	Signed ABN on file
-GO	Services provided by occupational therapist
-GP	Services provided by physical therapist
-GZ	No ABN on file
-KX	Used when services are *appropriately* provided in an episode that exceeds the therapy cap

NON-PAYABLE G Codes Guide for Functional Reporting

Code	Information Communicated	When Reported
GXXX	Current functional status	Therapy episode outset (initial eval) Reporting intervals (every 10th visit) Formal reeval (if performed during episode)
GXXX	Projected goal functional status	Therapy episode outset (initial eval) Reporting intervals (every 10th visit) Discharge from therapy OR to end reporting
GXXX	Discharge functional status	Discharge from therapy OR to end reporting

Continued

NON-PAYABLE G Codes Guide for Functional Reporting—cont'd

Mobility: Walking & Moving Around

G8984	Carrying, moving, & handling objects functional limitation, current status, at therapy episode outset, & at reporting intervals
G8985	Carrying, moving, & handling objects functional limitation, projected goal status, at therapy episode outset, at reporting intervals, & at discharge or to end reporting
G8986	Carrying, moving, & handling objects functional limitation, discharge status, at discharge from therapy or to end reporting

Changing & Maintaining Body Position

G8987	Self-care functional limitation, current status, at therapy episode outset, & at reporting intervals
G8988	Self-care functional limitation, projected goal status, at therapy episode outset, at reporting intervals, & at discharge or to end reporting
G8989	Self-care functional limitation, discharge status, at discharge from therapy, or to end reporting

Carrying, Moving, & Handling Objects

G8984	Carrying, moving, & handling objects functional limitation, current status, at therapy episode outset, & at reporting intervals
G8985	Carrying, moving, & handling objects functional limitation, projected goal status, at therapy episode outset, at reporting intervals, & at discharge or to end reporting
G8986	Carrying, moving, & handling objects functional limitation, discharge status, at discharge from therapy or to end reporting

Self Care

G8987	Self-care functional limitation, current status, at therapy episode outset, & at reporting intervals
G8988	Self-care functional limitation, projected goal status, at therapy episode outset, at reporting intervals, & at discharge or to end reporting
G8989	Self-care functional limitation, discharge status, at discharge from therapy or to end reporting

NON-PAYABLE G Codes Guide for Functional Reporting—cont'd

Other PT/OT Primary Functional Limitation

G8990	Other physical or occupational primary functional limitation, current status, at therapy episode outset, & at reporting intervals
G8991	Other physical or occupational primary functional limitation, projected goal status, at therapy episode outset, at reporting intervals, & at discharge or to end reporting
G8992	Other physical or occupational primary functional limitation, discharge status, at discharge from therapy or to end reporting

Other PT/OT Subsequent Functional Limitation

G8993	Other physical or occupational subsequent functional limitation, current status, at therapy episode outset, & at reporting intervals
G8994	Other physical or occupational subsequent functional limitation, projected goal status, at therapy episode outset, at reporting intervals, & at discharge or to end reporting
G8995	Other physical or occupational subsequent functional limitation, discharge status, & at discharge from therapy or to end reporting

Severity Modifiers

CH	0% impaired, limited or restricted
CI	At least 1% but less than 20% impaired, limited, or restricted
CJ	At least 20% but less than 40% impaired, limited, or restricted
CK	At least 40% but less than 60% impaired, limited, or restricted
CL	At least 60% but less than 80% impaired, limited, or restricted
CM	At least 80% but less than 100% impaired, limited, or restricted
CN	100% impaired, limited, or restricted

General Principles of "Best Practice" Documentation

Principles	Documentation Details
Consistent w/payer rules & regulations	**Medicare:** Know local coverage determination (LCD or LMRP). Know **terminology** used: • Medically necessary • Skilled • Qualified provider • Supervision • Practice setting **Commercial payers:** Review coverage: contact specific payers for details
Provides necessary detail pertaining to pt/client's condition	Answer question: "Why does pt/client need these services?" Physician referral w/diagnosis Rehab exam including: • Subjective info: Sx, impact on daily life & function • Objective info: impairments, functional limitations, & disability
Includes health-care provider's assessment of need for rehab service	Answer question: "How will pt/client benefit from service & how will service be administered?" Define "needs" for skilled services Identify measurable goals w/time frames, functional in nature & based on objective data
Outlines a detailed plan of care specific for individual pt/client	Specific modality/exercises w/frequency, duration, & extent of monitoring or supervision Individualized
Provides detail of interventions delivered	Includes specific interventions, responses to interventions, & progress toward goals Services provided billed appropriately
Describes a prognosis, w/a time frame & expected outcomes	Relate to PT diagnosis & reflect need for skilled care

SOAP NOTE Format

Component	Specific Details Included in Component
Subjective	Problem: chief complaint Information reported by pt/client related to management: • Pain or pain behavior • Current medications • Home situation • Past medical history • Prior level of functioning • Pt/client's goals • Current level of function
Objective	Past medical Hx from medical record Results of objective measurements/observations Description of any treatment provided Description of pt/client education provided Documentation of communication w/any other referrals/disciplines/MD
Assessment	Assessment of pt/client's problems for other health professionals to understand, overview of problems, & need for skilled intervention, to include: • Problem list • Goals: long-term (end of therapy) & short-term (interim) • Measurable, realistic, observable, time span, functional • Summary including practice pattern: PT impression including diagnosis & prognosis (guidance terminology)
Plan	• Frequency per d/wk • Treatment to be given • Education • Equipment needs • Plans for further assessment/referral • Criteria for discharge

Defensible Documentation*

Top 10 Tips

1. Limit use of abbreviations
2. Date and sign all entries
3. Document legibly
4. Report functional progress toward goals regularly
5. Document at the time of the visit when possible
6. Clearly identify note types, e.g., progress reports, daily notes
7. Include all related communications
8. Include missed/cancelled visits
9. Demonstrate skilled care and medical necessity
10. Demonstrate discharge planning throughout the episode of care

Documentation of Skilled Care

- Document clinical decision-making/problem-solving process
- Indicate why you chose the interventions/why they are necessary
- Document interventions connected to the impairment and functional limitation
- Document interventions connected to goals stated in plan of care
- Identify who is providing care (PT, PTA, or both)
- Document complications of comorbidities, safety issues, etc

Documenting Medical Necessity

- Services are consistent with nature and severity of illness, injury, and medical needs
- Services are specific, safe, and effective according to accepted medical practice
- There should be a reasonable expectation that observable and measurable improvement in functional ability will occur
- Services do not just promote the general welfare of the patient/client

*From APTA Defensible Documentation.

Common Abbreviations

AAA	abdominal aortic aneurysm
AAROM	active assisted range of motion
ABG	arterial blood gas
ACE	angiotensin-converting enzyme
ACLS	advanced cardiac life support
ACS	acute coronary syndrome
ADHD	attention-deficit hyperactivity disorder
ADL	activities of daily living
AED	automatic external defibrillator
AF	atrial fibrillation
AICD	automatic implantable cardiac defibrillator
AIDS	acquired immunodeficiency syndrome
AKA	above the knee amputation
ALS	amyotrophic lateral sclerosis
AMA	against medical advice
AMI	acute myocardial infarction
ANS	autonomic nervous system
ARC	AIDS-related complex
ARDS	acute respiratory distress syndrome
AROM	active range of motion
ASA	aspirin
ASD	atrial septal defect
AV	arteriovenous/atrioventricular
AVR	aortic valve repair
BBB	blood-brain barrier/bundle branch block
BCC	basal cell carcinoma
BE	barium enema
Bid	twice a day
BiPAP	bilevel positive airway pressure
BiVAD	biventricular assist device
BKA	below the knee amputation
BM	bowel movement
BMR	basal metabolic rate
BP	blood pressure
BRP	bathroom privileges
BS	blood sugar
BSA	body surface area
Bx	biopsy
CA	cancer

CABG	coronary artery bypass graft
CAD	coronary artery disease
CAPD	continuous abdominal peritoneal dialysis
Cc	chief complaint
CCU	coronary/critical care unit
CF	cystic fibrosis
CHF	congestive heart failure
CMV	cytomegalovirus
COPD/COLD	chronic obstructive pulmonary (lung) disease
CP	chest pain/cerebral palsy
CPAP	continuous positive airway pressure
CSF	cerebrospinal fluid
CVP	central venous pressure
CXR	chest x-ray
DIC	disseminated intravascular coagulation
DJD	degenerative joint disease
DM	diabetes mellitus
DNR	do not resuscitate
DOE	dyspnea on exertion
DTs	delirium tremors
DTR	deep tendon reflex
ECG	electrocardiogram
ECT	electroconvulsive therapy
ED	erectile dysfunction
EENT	eye, ear, nose, & throat
EPS	electrophysiology study
ET	endotracheal tube
ETOH	alcohol
FHR	fetal heart rate
GCS	Glasgow Coma Scale
GDM	gestational diabetes mellitus
GERD	gastroesophageal reflux disease
GFR	glomerular filtration rate
GSW	gunshot wound
HA	headache
HAV	hepatitis A virus
HBV	hepatitis B virus
HOH	hard of hearing
HTN	hypertension
Hx	history
IABP	intraaortic balloon pump

ICP	intracranial pressure
IDDM	insulin-dependent diabetes mellitus
JVD	jugular venous distention
KUB	kidney, ureters, and bladder
LFT	liver function test
LLL	left lower lobe
LLQ	left lower quadrant
LOC	loss of consciousness
LVAD	left ventricular assist device
MAP	mean arterial pressure
MRSA	methicillin-resistant *Staphylococcus aureus*
MVA	motor vehicle accident
MVR	mitral valve replacement
NEB	nebulized
NIDDM	non-insulin dependent diabetes
NKA	no known allergies
NPO	nothing by mouth
NSR	normal sinus rhythm
NWB	non-weight-bearing
OD	overdose
ORIF	open reduction internal fixation
PCA	patient/client controlled anesthesia
PCWP	pulmonary capillary wedge pressure
PE	pulmonary embolus
PEA	pulseless electrical activity
PICC	peripherally inserted central catheter
PKU	phenylketonuria
PMH	past medical history
PND	paroxysmal nocturnal dyspnea
PRN	as needed
PROM	passive range of motion
PWB	partial weight-bearing
RICE	rest, ice, compression, elevation
RLQ	right lower quadrant
RR	recovery room/respiratory rate
S & S	signs and symptoms
SIDS	sudden infant death syndrome
SLP	speech language pathology
SNF	skilled nursing facility
SOB	shortness of breath
STD	sexually transmitted disease

Sz	seizure
Sx	symptoms
TCA	tricyclic antidepressant
TIA	transient ischemic attack
TMJ	temporomandibular joint
TPN	total parenteral nutrition
TTWB	toe touch weight-bearing
TURP	transurethral resection prostatectomy
UTI	urinary tract infection
VQ scan	ventilation-perfusion scan
VRE	vancomycin-resistant enterococcus
WPW	Wolff-Parkinson-White

Red Flags

Assessment of these areas should raise concern whether the problem has a systemic or viscerogenic origin.

Past Medical Hx
- Personal/family Hx of cancer
- Recent infection when followed by neurological Sx, joint or back pain
- Recent Hx of trauma
- Hx of immunosuppression
- Hx of drug use: injection

Risk Factors of Possible Systemic Disease
- Substance abuse including alcohol, drug, or tobacco
- Age
- Gender
- BMI
- Exposure to radiation
- Race/ethnicity
- Sedentary lifestyle
- Domestic violence
- Hysterectomy
- Occupation

Clinical Presentation
- Insidious onset/unknown etiology
- Sx not improved or relieved by physical therapy
- Significant weight loss or gain without attempting to lose or gain
- Gradual, progressive, or cyclical presentation of Sx
- Sx that are unrelieved by rest or change of position
- Sx persisting beyond expected time of condition
- Sx do not fit typical neuromuscular or musculoskeletal pattern
- A growing mass or a hematoma that is not decreasing in size
- Postmenopausal bleeding
- Bilateral Sx such as edema, numbness, tingling, clubbing, nail bed changes, skin rash, or pigment changes
- Change in muscle tone or ROM in those with neurological conditions

Pain Pattern
- Pain w/full painless ROM
- Pain not consistent with psychological overlay
- Throbbing or deep, aching pain

- Poorly localized pain
- Pain that comes and goes like spasms
- Pain associated with S&S relating to certain viscera or system, e.g., GI, GU, cardiac, pulmonary
- Change of pain with food intake

Associated S&S
- Unusual menstrual cycle or Sx
- Presence of unusual/abnormal vital signs, including HR, temp, etc
- Proximal muscle weakness and/or DTRs
- Change in mental status including confusion
- Joint pain with skin rashes

Cancer Assessment

Early Warning Cancer Signs (American Cancer Society)

- Changes in bowel/bladder habits
- Sore that does not heal in 6 wk
- Unusual bleeding or discharge
- Thickening or lump in breast or elsewhere
- Indigestion or difficulty in swallowing
- Obvious change in wart/mole
- Nagging cough or hoarseness
- Proximal muscle weakness
- Change in deep tendon reflexes

Other Screening Clues

- Previous personal Hx of any cancer
- Recent wt loss of 10 lb or more within 1 mo
- Constant pain, unrelieved by rest or change in position
- Night pain
- Development of new neurological deficits
- Changes in size, shape, tenderness, & consistency of lymph nodes, painless & present in >1 location
- Women: chest, breast, axillary, or shoulder pain of unknown cause
- Bloody sputum

Adapted from Goodman C. and Snyder T. *Differential Diagnosis for Physical Therapists*, ed. 4. Philadelphia: Elsevier, 2006. p. 7.

Types of Cancer

Type	Etiology/Location
Adenocarcinoma	Glandular tissue
Carcinoma	Epithelial tissue
Glioma	Brain, supportive tissue, spinal cord
Leukemia	Blood-forming cells
Lymphoma	Lymphatic cells
Melanoma	Pigment cells
Myeloma	Plasma cells
Sarcoma	Mesenchymal cells

Cancer Staging (TNM)*

Tumor (T)	Node (N)	Metastasis (M)
T1 = small, confined	N0 = no other involvement	M0 = no metastasis
T2–T3 = medium	N1–N3 = moderate involvement	M1 = metastasis
T4 = large	N4 = extensive	

*Most types of cancer have TNM designations.

Other Cancer Staging

Type of Cancer	Staging
Brain, spinal cord	Cell type and grade
Blood/bone marrow	No clear-cut staging system
Lymphomas	Ann Arbor staging classification
Cervix, uterus, ovary, vagina, vulva	IFGO staging system

Ann Arbor Staging Classification for Lymphomas

Stage	Distribution of Disease
I	Single lymph node region or single extralymphatic organ or site involved
II	≥2 lymph node regions on same side of diaphragm involved or involvement of limited continuous extralymphatic organs
III	Lymph node regions on both sides of diaphragm, limited contiguous extralymphatic organ involvement, or both
IV	Multiple, disseminated involvement of one or more extralymphatic organs with or without lymphatic involvement

Adapted from Carbone PP et al. Report of the Committee on Hodgkin's Disease Staging Classification. Cancer Res 1971;31(11):1860–1.

Summary Staging

Summary staging groups cancer cases into five main categories.

In situ—Abnormal cells are present only in the layer of cells in which they developed.

Localized—Cancer is limited to the organ in which it began, without evidence of spread.

Regional—Cancer has spread beyond the primary site to nearby lymph nodes or organs and tissues.

Distant—Cancer has spread from the primary site to distant organs or distant lymph nodes.

Unknown—There is not enough information to determine the stage.

Grading of Neoplasms

Grade	Characteristics
Grade 1	Tumor cells resemble original tissue.
Grades II and III	Tumor cells do not resemble original tissue and are moderately differentiated.
Grade IV	Tumor cells are poorly differentiated (anaplastic). Origin of cell is difficult to determine.

Testing for Cancer Staging

- Physical exam
- Laboratory tests
- Pathology reports
- Surgical reports
- Imaging studies: produce pictures of areas inside the body

Common Side Effects of Radiation Therapy

- Skin reactions/slow wound healing
- Limb edema
- Contractures, fibrosis
- Alopecia
- Neuropathies
- Brain: seizures, visual disturbances, headaches
- Bone marrow suppression
- Pulmonary: cough, pneumonitis, pulmonary fibrosis
- GI: esophagitis, nausea, vomiting, diarrhea
- GU: cystitis, urinary frequency

Precautions to Take With Radiation Therapy

- Defer PT while patient/client has radiation seeds
- Massage, heat not indicated for area radiated for 1 yr
- Promote ROM to prevent contracture for months following radiation
- Areas marked in blue (EBRT radiation) or black (maximal dosage) should be treated cautiously, as skin will be fragile
- Monitor for nausea/vomiting despite being treated with antiemetics; these may not be effective and nutrition is important

Precautions With Chemotherapy

- Monitor vital signs always, especially with the more toxic chemo agents as side effects affect heart, lungs, and CNS
- Monitor lab values, especially neutropenia and absolute neutrophil count (ANC). Patient/clients may be on isolation
- Some agents are extremely toxic and patient/clients must remain in room to avoid risk to other patient/clients/health-care workers. Check if unsure

- Delay or modify therapy until side effects from chemotherapy are minimized or alleviated
- Chemotherapy can affect appetite and nutrition. Work with dietitian to ensure adequate nutrition for strengthening and conditioning
- Provide emotional support when patient/client unable to participate in rehab due to side effects of chemotherapy
- All patient/clients require aerobic conditioning when they can tolerate it. Begin with intervals and build up the time involved
- Keep in mind patients may continue to experience side effects for years or develop side effects years after initial chemotherapy

Est. New Cancer Cases: 10 Leading Sites by Sex, United States 2005

Men	% of Cases	Women	% of Cases
Prostate	33	Breast	32
Lung & bronchus	13	Lung & bronchus	12
Colon & rectum	10	Colon & rectum	11
Urinary bladder	7	Uterine carpus	6
Melanoma of skin	5	Non-Hodgkin lymphoma	4
Non-Hodgkin lymphoma	4	Melanoma of skin	4
Kidney & renal pelvis	3	Ovary	3
Leukemia	3	Thyroid	3
Oral cavity & pharynx	3	Urinary bladder	2
Pancreas	2	Pancreas	2
All other sites	17	All other sites	21

Cancer Deaths by Site, United States 2005

Men	% of Cases	Women	% of Cases
Lung & bronchus	31	Lung & bronchus	27
Prostate	10	Breast	15
Colon & rectum	10	Colon & rectum	10
Pancreas	5	Ovary	6
Leukemia	4	Pancreas	6
Esophagus	4	Leukemia	4
Liver & intrahepatic bile duct	3	Non-Hodgkin lymphoma	3
Non-Hodgkin lymphoma	3	Uterine carpus	3
Urinary bladder	3	Multiple myeloma	2
Kidney & renal pelvis	3	Brain & other nervous system	2
All other sites	24	All other sites	22

Diabetes Assessment

Characteristics	Type I	Type II*
Onset	In childhood or young adulthood	Adult onset, >40 yr
Etiology	Little or no insulin production by beta cells of islet of Langerhans	Partial ↓ of insulin production or ↓ sensitivity of tissues to insulin
Treatment	Insulin-dependent	Noninsulin-dependent, may be controlled w/diet, exercise, & wt loss

*Type II diabetics often become like type I diabetics because they become insulin dependent. This happens over time when patient/clients do not follow diet and exercise and pathological changes occur to pancreas (shrinking) with less insulin production resulting.

Systems Affected by Diabetes

System	Impairments & Abnormalities	Implications for Rehab Professionals
Cardiovascular	↑BP Impairment in circulation in extremities & small vessels Silent ischemia/silent MI	Monitor BP at rest & w/activity Evaluate any wounds Monitor Sx w/activity; look for SOB: NOT angina
Endocrine	↑Cholesterol ↑Triglycerides	Evaluate lab results; referral to control lipids
Integumentary	Impaired healing due to impaired circulation	Evaluate skin; assess postsurgical scars/incisions
Nervous	Peripheral neuropathies ↓Sensation in hands & feet ↓Sensation of chest pain Autonomic neuropathies Orthostatic hypotension ABN VS responses	Instruct in skin checks, foot care, & good footwear SOB = angina in diabetics/ may not perceive typical angina Monitor VS w/all activities
Ophthalmic	Retinopathies: poor vision	Assess visual
Renal	Renal artery disease; impaired function of glomerulus, impaired filtering	Rule out kidney problems by evaluating labs (creat & BUN)

Signs/Symptoms of Hypoglycemia

Adrenergic*	Neuroglucopenic
Weakness	Headache
Sweating	Hypothermia
Tachycardia	Visual disturbances
Palpitations	Mental dullness
Tremor	Confusion
Nervousness	Amnesia
Irritability	Seizures

Signs/Symptoms of Hypoglycemia—cont'd

Adrenergic*	Neuroglucopenic
Tingling mouth & fingers	Coma
Hunger	
Nausea	
Vomiting	

*These symptoms will not be visible or present with beta blockers.

Exercise Considerations for Diabetics

- Type of insulin used
- Onset of effect of insulin
- Peak effect of insulin
- Length of insulin effect
- Injection site
- Time between insulin taken & onset of exercise
- Time between exercise & last meal

Differentiation of Osteoarthritis & Rheumatoid Arthritis

	Osteoarthritis	Rheumatoid Arthritis
Cause	Breakdown of joint cartilage ↑ w/age & w/specific joint injury/trauma	Autoimmune cause Possible genetic predisposition
Pain origin	Bone-on-bone rubbing in joint causes pain	Inflammation of synovium in joint
Joint(s)	Begins in a single joint	Multiple joints are involved
Sx	Pain w/repetitive use in affected joint(s) AM stiffness (<30 min), joint pain worsens as day progresses Stiffness worsens with prolonged inactivity	AM stiffness >1 hr Redness/warmth Involvement of small bones of hands & feet Extreme fatigue Symmetrical joint involvement

Continued

Differentiation of Osteoarthritis & Rheumatoid Arthritis—cont'd

	Osteoarthritis	Rheumatoid Arthritis
Diagnosis	Physical exam, Sx Arthrocentesis & joint fluid removal	Labs: + rheumatoid factor Anti CCP test Elevated C reactive protein Erythrocyte sed rate
Treatment	Pain relief, restore function NSAIDs, analgesics, steroid injections Support/bracing, strengthening of muscles around joint, weight reduction	Medications: biologics, DMARDs, corticosteroids, NSAIDs Resting of inflamed joints, splinting Last resort is surgery

Effects of Aging

Tissue/Organ	Aging Changes
Skeletal tissue	Decline in bone mineral beginning in 30s ↑ risk of osteopenia ↑ risk of osteoporosis
Body composition	Shift to ↓ lean mass & ↑ fat mass ↑ intrabdominal fat
Collagenous tissues	Loss of water from matrix, ↑ in crosslinks, loss of elastic fibers.
Cardiovascular tissues	Decline in maximum heart rate Decline in VO_2 max Stiffer, less compliant vascular tissues Slower ventricle filling time with reduced cardiac output Loss of cells from the SA node Reduced arteriovenous O_2 uptake
Nervous system	Slowing of movement speed
Immune system	Decreased immunity
Hormones	Decreased functioning of hormones, increase in dysfunction

Recommended Daily Nutrition

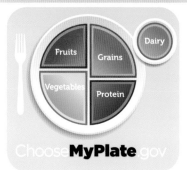

Choose My Plate

From the United States Dept. of Agriculture http://www.choosemyplate.gov/

Daily Dietary Recommendations From Joint WHO/FAO Expert Consultation 2002

Dietary Factor	Recommendations
Total fat	15%–30%
Saturated fatty acids	<10%
Polyunsaturated fatty acids	6%–10%
Trans fatty acids	<1%
Total carbohydrates	55%–75%
Free sugars	<10%
Complex carbohydrates	No recommendation
Proteins	10%–15%
Cholesterol	<300 mg
Fruits & vegetables	>400 g/d
Sodium	<5 g/d

ICD-10 Codes for Cardiovascular and Pulmonary Dysfunction

(I 00–I 99) Diseases of the Circulatory System

I00–I02	Acute rheumatic fever
I05–I09	Chronic rheumatic heart diseases
I10–I15	Hypertensive diseases
I20–I25	Ischemic heart diseases
I26–I28	Pulmonary heart disease and diseases of pulmonary circulation
I30–I52	Other forms of heart disease
I60–I69	Cerebrovascular diseases
I70–I79	Diseases of arteries, arterioles, and capillaries
I80–I89	Diseases of veins, lymphatic vessels, and lymph nodes; not elsewhere classified
I95–I99	Other and unspecified disorders of circulatory system

(J00–J99) Diseases of the Respiratory System

J00–J06	Acute upper respiratory infections
J09–J18	Influenza and pneumonia
J20–J22	Other acute lower respiratory infections
J30–J39	Other diseases of upper respiratory tract
J40–J47	Chronic lower respiratory diseases
J60–J70	Lung diseases due to external agents
J80–J84	Other respiratory diseases principally affecting interstitium
J85–J86	Suppurative and necrotic conditions of lower respiratory tract
J90–J94	Other diseases of pleura
J95–J99	Other diseases of respiratory system

R00–R09 Symptoms and Signs Involving the Circulatory and Respiratory Systems

R00	Abnormalities of heart beat
R01	Cardiac murmurs and other cardiac sounds
R03	Elevated blood-pressure reading, without diagnosis
R04	Hemorrhage from respiratory passages
R05	Cough
R06	Abnormalities of breathing
R07	Pain in throat and chest
R09	Other symptoms and signs involving the circulatory and respiratory systems

From World Health Organization. International Statistical Classification of Diseases, ed. 10. http://apps.who.int/classifications/icd10/browse/2010/en with permission.

Quick Screen for Cardiovascular & Pulmonary Dysfunction

Eval/Screen	Results	NL/ABN
Heart sounds		
Lung sounds		
Vital signs		
Symptoms		
Diagnostics:		
ECG		
Echo		
CXR		
PFT		
ABGs		
VQ scan/spiral CT		
Biopsy		
Other		
Labs:		
Chol/TG		
Troponin, CPK-MB, LDH-1		
Glucose, HbA$_1$C		
BUN, creatinine		
BNP		
Other ABN lab results?		
Meds: What are they & what are they used for?		

Cardiac Anatomy

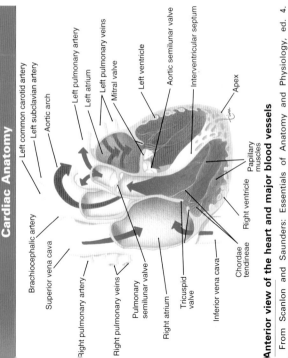

Left common carotid artery
Left subclavian artery
Aortic arch
Left pulmonary artery
Left atrium
Left pulmonary veins
Mitral valve
Left ventricle
Aortic semilunar valve
Interventricular septum
Apex
Papillary muscles
Right ventricle
Chordae tendineae
Inferior vena cava
Tricuspid valve
Right atrium
Pulmonary semilunar valve
Right pulmonary veins
Right pulmonary artery
Superior vena cava
Brachiocephalic artery

Anterior view of the heart and major blood vessels

From Scanlon and Saunders: Essentials of Anatomy and Physiology, ed. 4. Philadelphia, F.A. Davis Co., 2003, p 262.

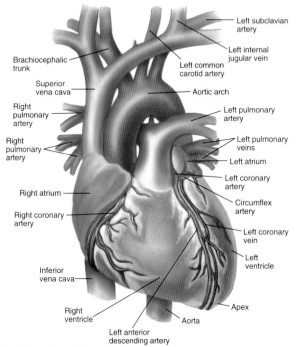

Frontal section of the heart.

From Gylys: Medical Terminology Systems: A Body Systems Approach, ed. 5. Philadelphia, F.A. Davis Co., 2003, p 191.

Lung Anatomy

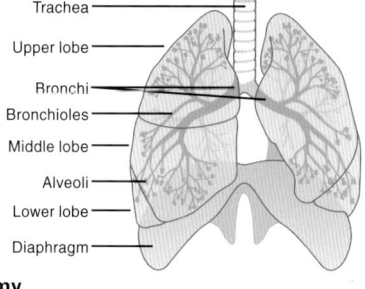

Trachea

Upper lobe

Bronchi

Bronchioles

Middle lobe

Alveoli

Lower lobe

Diaphragm

Lung anatomy.

Pulmonary Assessment

Evaluation of Breathing

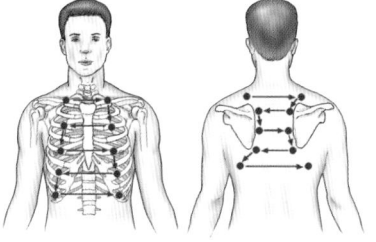

Anterior view

Posterior view

Auscultation.

Errors of auscultation to avoid:

- Listening to breath sounds through patient/client's gown
- Allowing tubing to rub against bed rails or gown

- Attempting to listen in a noisy room
- Interpreting chest hair sounds as adventitious lung sounds
- Auscultating only the "convenient" areas (eg, only anterior)

Palpation of Chest Wall

ABN FINDINGS & INTERPRETATION

- Shift to "affected side": ↓ lung tissue
  (lobectomy, pneumonectomy)
- Shift to "unaffected side":
- ↑ pressure on lung (large pleural effusion)
- Lack of symmetry between sides: area not
  moving equal to opposite side

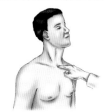

Palpation for presence/absence of tracheal deviation.

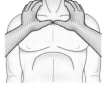 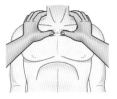

Palpation of upper lobe motion.

From White, G. *Respiratory Notes*, Philadelphia: F.A. Davis, 2008.

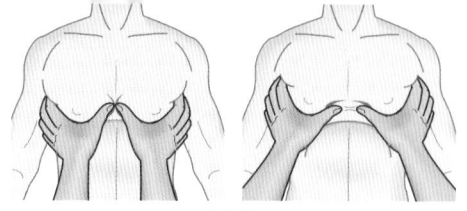

Anterior

Palpation of right middle and left lingual lobe motion.

From White, G. *Respiratory Notes,* Philadelphia: F.A. Davis, 2008.

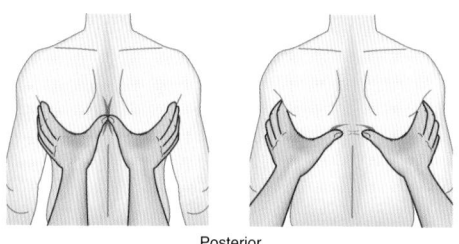

Posterior

Palpation of lower lobe motion.

From White, G. *Respiratory Notes,* Philadelphia: F.A. Davis, 2008.

■ ↑ muscle activity of scalenes: ↑ accessory muscle use; lack of diaphragmatic movement found in COPD, spinal cord injury, scarring, or improper breathing mechanics.

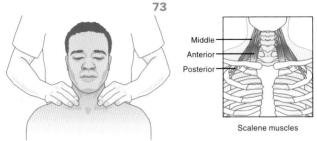

Middle
Anterior
Posterior

Scalene muscles

Palpation of scalene muscle activity with breathing.

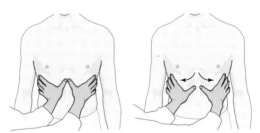

Palpation of diaphragmatic motion.

- Normally, palpation reveals uniform vibration throughout
- ↑ Vibration indicates secretions
- ↓ Fremitus indicates ↑ in air

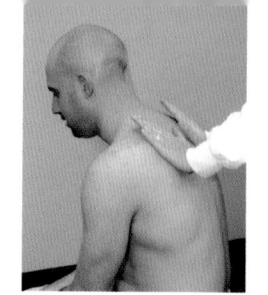

Palpation for fremitus (using heel of hand).

Rule out for angina pain:

- ↑ pain over bone indicates fracture
- ↑ pain over muscle may be muscle inflammation due to overuse or injury
- ↑ discomfort w/deep inspiration or palpation is non-anginal
- Pain at costochondral junctions could be joint inflammation

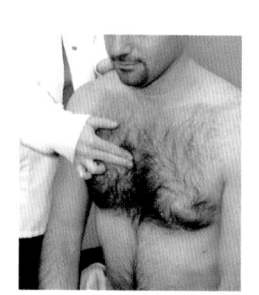

Palpation for chest wall pain or discomfort.

Assessment of Breath Sounds

Breath Sounds	Interpretation
Adequate sound, pitch, intensity on inspir & expir: no ABN sounds	NL
↓ sounds	Hyperinflated lungs: COPD Hypoinflation: acute lung disease (eg, atelectasis, pneumothorax, pleural effusion)
Absent sounds	Pleural effusion, pneumothorax, obesity, 3rd trimester pregnancy in lower lobes, severe hyperinflation as in COPD
Bronchial breath sounds	Consolidation (pneumonia), large atelectasis w/patent airway adjacent
Wheezes (rhonchi)	Diffuse airway obstruction usually associated w/bronchospasm or tumor OR localized stenosis
Crackles (rales)	Secretions present if on inspir & expir; atelectasis if on inspir only
↓ voice sounds (repeating 99 or A)	Atelectasis, pleural effusion, pneumothorax
↑ voice sounds	Consolidation, pulmonary fibrosis
Extrapulmonary adventitious sound: pleural rub	Pleural inflammation or pleuritis

Assessment of Phonation, Cough, & Sputum

Assessments	ABN Findings & Interpretation	
Phonation	Dyspnea of phonation Count words expressed before next breath Poor voice control: weak musculature	
Cough	Ineffective: assess for weakness of musculature & pain Productive of secretions: evaluate secretions & chronicity of secretions Violent/spasmodic: may be aspiration or brochospasm Nonproductive but persistent: auscultate: assess for signs of infection, pulm fibrosis, pulm infiltrates	
Sputum	**Evaluate color:**	
	White/clear	Noninfected
	Yellow/green	Infection
	Blood tinged	Could be irritation of trachea/bronchial coughing
	Rust colored	TB or fungal infection
	Frank blood	Neoplastic or pulmonary infarct RED FLAG for treatment
	Evaluate consistency:	
	Thick, formerly mucoid	Acute/exacerbation, may also be dehydrated
	Frothy	Pulm edema/heart failure
	Evaluate amt:	
	Copious	Long-standing problem
	↑ from NL	Indicates acute exacerbation
	Evaluate smell:	
	Bronchiectasis	Infective
Sputum breath	Foul smelling: anaerobic infection of mouth/respiratory tract Acetone: ketoacidosis	

Assessment of Assisted Breathing

Modes of O_2 Delivery

- FIO_2 = fraction of inspired oxygen
  - % of inhaled air that is oxygen
  - Room air = 21% O_2

Oxygen given via nasal cannula:

- 1 L/min 24%
- 2 L/min 28%
- 3 L/min 32%
- 4 L/min 36%
- 5 L/min 40%
- 6 L/min 44%

Delivery Mode	Indications, Limitations, Constraints
Flowmeter	O_2 provided by institution from wall; use acute care & high flow rates NOT portable; ↑ mobility w/tubing & nasal cannula or mask
Nasal cannula	Use w/O_2 at flow rates of 1–6 L/min; provides FIO_2 of 24%–44% No benefit if NOT breathing through nose
High-flow nasal cannula	Best for patient/clients needing >6 L/min NC; highest % O_2 up to 75% FIO_2 at 15 L/min; more comfortable, can eat/drink/talk more easily than w/mask New to many clinics
Oxymyzer	Specialized NC w/O_2 reservoir; conserves O_2; uses 25%–75% less O_2; ↓ O_2 needed by patient/client, ↑ savings of O_2; good way to deliver O_2 at home
O_2 concentrator; H-cylinder	Contains 6900 L O_2; use at home or w/high flow rates Big: not portable
O_2 cylinders	Most widely used Heavy, wt: 17 lb; hard to use & also has mobility problems; vol ↓ at high flow

Continued

Delivery Mode	Indications, Limitations, Constraints
Portable liquid O_2 unit	More lightweight for portable use; can be delivered pulsed or continuous flow. Continuous flow best for endurance activities (walking, etc) Wt: <4 lb; empties fast w/high flow; if on pulsed mode, conserves O_2 use but patient/clients may not perform as well w/endurance activities
Portable oxygen concentrator	Lightweight (wt <10 lb); portable; allows for longer use of liquid O_2; 1050 mL/min oxygen capacity; 8 h battery life
Simple mask	Delivery of O_2 over face w/humid air at ↑ flow rates (5–10 L/min); provides FIO_2 35%–55% Claustrophobic w/mask, difficult to talk; best for mouth breather
Aerosol mask	For controlled % of O_2 at flow rates >10–12 L/min; FIO_2 35%–100% Mask not tolerated by patient/client for long periods
Venturi mask	Provides greater flow of gas w/use of room air through side port (4–10 L/min); FIO_2 24%–50% (see Venturi Valves Color Guide box below) Mask not tolerated by patient/client for long periods
Partial nonrebreather mask	Mask w/an O_2 reservoir (bag) that provides a higher amount of O_2 to patient/client NRB flow: 6 L/min = 60% 7 L/min = 70% 8–10 L/min = 80+% Advantage: requires ↓ flow of O_2 for FIO_2 needed
CPAP	Continuous positive airway pressure used to ↓ airway closure, improve sleep apnea as well as patient/clients demonstrating poor ABGs w/sleeping

Venturi Valves: Color Guide		
Color	**Flow Rate (L/min)**	**O_2 Delivered (%)**
Blue	2	24
White	4	28
Yellow	6	35
Red	8	40
Green	12	60
Treatment w/O_2	60% or >101 rebreathing	90–94

Oxygen Use

Current recommendations for use of O_2 short-term from ATS:

- In presence of PaO_2 <55 mm Hg or SpO_2 <88%
- When PaO_2 ≥55 mm Hg but ≤ 59 mm Hg & add'l diagnoses (PAH, cor pulmonale)
- When PaO_2 ≥60 mm Hg or SpO_2 ≥90% and desaturates during activity, individuals should use O_2 w/all activities
- Titrate O_2 w/all activities to keep SpO_2 >90%
- Reduce O_2 at rest
- Assess O_2 w/sleeping as well as activity

Errors in Use of Pulse Oximetry

- Low perfusion (CO) or arrhythmias
- Incorrect probe—may benefit from head probe
- Fingernail polish, dirt affecting sensor light path
- Cold temperature—shunting of blood from extremity
- Wrong finger placement—use 3rd or 4th finger
- Motion or weight-bearing

Kim 2008; Proc Am Thor Soc.

Mechanical Ventilation/Assisted Ventilation

Modes	Indications
Controlled vent: + pressure breaths at a set rate	To control rate, depth, & frequency of every breath
Assist or assist-control vent: + pressure breaths at a set rate unless patient/client triggers machine w/neg inspir force < preset threshold force	Patient/client controls ventilation, but ↓ inspir vol; used for post-op care, weaning, to avoid ↑ peak airway pressure; patient/client difficult to manage w/o sedation/paralyzing meds
IMV: preset rate, spontaneous efforts +/– SIMV: mandatory breath initiated by spontaneous inspir effort	Patient/client can breathe spontaneously through ventilator circuit, but ventilator imposes mandatory breaths at preset intervals; SIMV delivers ↓ VT w/↑ airway pressure
PSV: patient/client's spontaneous vent efforts PLUS preset amt of pressure	Reduces work of breathing. Used for post-op care, weaning, to avoid high peak airway pressure; patient/clients difficult to manage w/o sedation/paralyzing drugs
Nasal CPAP	Treatment for obstructive sleep apnea; noninvasive ventilation
BiPap or bilevel positive airway pressure	Noninvasive vent: improves ventilation & VS w/acute pulmonary edema; works more rapidly than CPAP; different pressures on inspiration and expir
Vent: augmentation/ modifications 1. Inspiratory hold 2. PEEP 3. Expiratory retard 4. CPAP	1. Preset pressure or vol held for a set time before exhalation permitted. Used to ↓ atelectasis 2. Resistance after exhalation to keep alveoli open longer; recruits collapsed alveoli 3. Resistance applied to exhalation 4. Provides ↑ baseline pressure when patient/client breathing spontaneously

Adaptive Equipment Checklist

ICU or Med/Surg Room

Monitoring/Care Equipment	Present	Absent
Oxygen		
O$_2$ saturation monitor		
Telemetry		
IV lines		
Arterial line		
Suction		
NG/feeding tube		
Intra-aortic balloon pump		
ECMO		
Ventilator		
Other:		

Cardiovascular Assessment

Heart Sounds

Sound	NL or ABN	Definition
S$_1$ (LUB)	NL	Associated w/closure of mitral & tricuspid valves; associated w/onset of systole; loudest in mitral and tricuspid areas
S$_2$ (DUB)	NL	Associated w/closure of pulmonic & aortic valves; associated w/onset of vent diastole; loudest at aortic or pulmonic regions
S$_4$ (LA Lub Dub)	ABN	Auscultation w/bell of steth: atrial gallop; sign of ↑ resistance to vent filling. S$_4$ in: CAD, pulmonary disease, hypertensive heart disease, & post MI or CABG.

Continued

Sound	NL or ABN	Definition
Murmurs Grading: I–IV/VI	**ABN**	Indicate backflow or resistance through valves • I/VI inaudible w/o steth • IV–VI/VI very loud Systolic: heard between S_1 & S_2 Diastolic: heard after S_2
Pericardial Friction Rub		Squeaky/creaky leathery sound occurring w/each beat of heart. Indicates fluid in or inflammation of pericardial sac

Auscultation of Heart Sounds

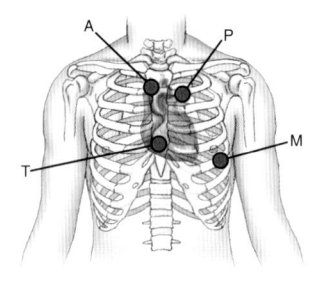

Assessment of Circulation

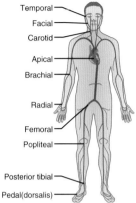

Temporal
Facial
Carotid
Apical
Brachial
Radial
Femoral
Popliteal
Posterior tibial
Pedal(dorsalis)

Assessment of circulation.

Tests for Arterial Insufficiency	
Tests	**Description**
Ankle Brachial Index (ABI): Noninvasive test for evaluating peripheral arterial disease	• Place pneumatic cuff around ankle above malleoli • Place Doppler ultrasound probe over posterior tibial artery; measure pressure at this site • Place Doppler probe over dorsalis pedis artery, measure pressure • NL pressures should differ no >10 mm Hg Pressure difference >15 mm Hg suggests proximal occlusion or stenosis

Continued

Tests for Arterial Insufficiency—cont'd

Tests	Description
Capillary Refill: Indicator of surface arterial blood flow	• Observe color of patient/client's toe • Push against distal tip of toe and hold for 5 sec • Record capillary refill time—amount of time required for toe surface color to return • Normal time is <3 sec
Rubor of Dependency: Indirectly assesses arterial flow in the lower extremity	• Patient/client positioned supine, note color of plantar aspect of foot • Elevate lower extremity to 60° for 1 min • Note color of plantar surface of foot; normal = little to no change in color; arterial insufficiency = pale coloring • Return lower extremity to support surface • Record how long for original color to return; normal = 15–20 sec • Pallor after 45–60 sec of elevation = mild insufficiency • Pallor after 30–45 sec of elevation = moderate insufficiency • Pallor within 25 sec of elevation = severe insufficiency
Venous Filling Time	• Patient/client positioned supine, observe superficial veins on dorsal foot • Elevate limb to 60° for 1 min • Place limb in dependent position • Record time for superficial veins to refill • Normal = 5–15 sec; if >20 sec = severe arterial insufficiency; if refill occurs immediately = venous insufficiency

Assessment of Edema

1+	Barely perceptible depression (pit)
2+	Easily identified depress (EID) rebounds w/in 15 sec
3+	EID rebounds to original w/in 15–30 sec
4+	EID rebounds >30 sec

Assessment of Physiological Responses to Activity					
Activity	**HR**	**BP**	**Symptoms**	**SpO$_2$**	**RPE**
Supine					
Sit					
Stand					
Ambulation (include assistance needed, need for assistive device, feet walked)					
Performance of ADL					

Borg Scale

Can use for rating perceived exertion of tasks, or used as dyspnea scale rating amount of dyspnea w/task.

   6.
   7. Very, very light
   8.
   9. Very light
10.
11. Fairly light
12.
13. Somewhat hard
14.
15. Hard
16.
17. Very hard
18.
19. Very, very hard

Adapted from Borg, GA: Psychological basis of physical exertion. Med Sci Sports Exerc 14:377, 1982.

Resting Blood Pressure Guidelines NHLBI 2003

Stage	Systolic	Diastolic
Normal	<120	<80
Prehypertension	120–139	80–89
Stage 1 hypertension	140–159	90–99
Stage 2 hypertension	>160	>100

Physiological Responses to Activity

	NL	ABN	Notes
HR	**Resting:** 60–90 bpm adult; 50–100 bpm adolescent; 75–140 bpm child; 80–180 bpm infant **Activity:** Gradual rate of rise correlated w/intensity of activity **Steady state exercise:** No Δ rhythm should be regular	**Resting:** <60 bpm or >90 bpm **Activity:** Rapid rate of ↑ Little or no Δ w/↑ activity Irregular w/activity **Steady state exercise:** Progressive ↑	Athletes: RHR may be <60 Fever, anxiety, meds ↑ RHR Irregular at rest: check underlying rhythm; see ECG section
BP	**Resting:** Systolic <130 mm Hg; 70 mm Hg infant; 90 mm Hg child Diastolic <90 mm Hg; 55 mm Hg infant; 58 mm Hg child **Activity:** Systolic: progressive ↑ correlated w/intensity of exercise Diastolic: +/− 10 mm Hg **Steady state exercise:** No Δ in systolic or diastolic	**Resting:** Syst >140 or diast >90 **Activity:** Rapid ↑ in systolic Blunted rate of rise w/↑ activity ↓ Systolic w/↑ activity Progressive ↑ in diastolic **Steady state exercise:** Progressive ↑	↓ in systolic w/Δ in position (sit to stand) is orthostatic ↓ w/activity: exertional hypotension Compare standing w/ walking BP, NOT sitting to walking
SpO₂	**Resting:** 98%–100% **Activity:** No Δ	**Resting:** <98% **Activity:** ↓ w/↑ activity	Individuals Δ breathing rate when being observed Often counted while evaluating HR

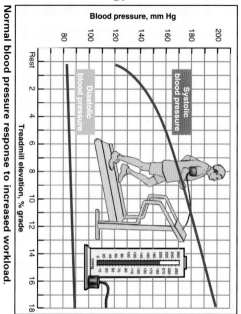

Blood pressure, mm Hg

Systolic blood pressure

Diastolic blood pressure

Treadmill elevation, % grade

Normal blood pressure response to increased workload.

Assessment of Angina Symptoms

- Many presenting Sx are subjective, such as:
    - extreme fatigue
    - lethargy
    - breathlessness
    - weakness
- Isolated pain in the right mid-biceps may delay diagnosis.

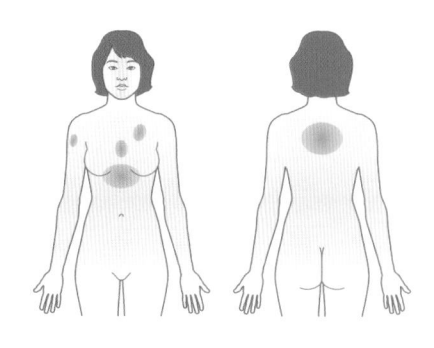

Pain patterns associated with angina in women.

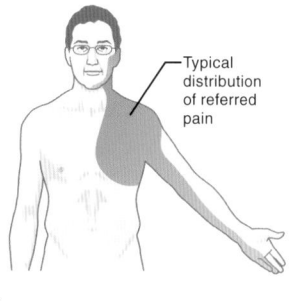

Typical distribution of referred pain

Pain patterns associated with angina in men.

Pain Patterns Associated With Angina

- Pain patterns in women may differ from patterns in men.
- Area of substernal discomfort projects to L shoulder & arm over the distribution of the ulnar nerve. (*left*)
- Referred pain may be present only in L shoulder or in shoulder & along arm only to elbow.
- Anginal pain may occasionally be referred to the back in area of L scapula or interscapular region. (*right*)
- Fatigue, weakness, or breathlessness

Scales for Assessment of Angina & Dyspnea

5-Grade Angina	5-Grade Dyspnea	Modified Borg
0. No angina	0. No dyspnea	0. Nothing
1. Light, barely noticeable	1. Mild, noticeable 2. Mild, some difficulty	1. Very slight 2. Slight
2. Moderate, bothersome	3. Moderate difficulty, but can continue	3. Moderate 4. Somewhat severe
3. Severe, very uncomfortable; pre-infarction pain	4. Severe difficulty, cannot continue	5. Severe 6. 7. Very severe
4. Most pain ever experienced; infarction pain		8. 9. 10. Extremely severe; maximal

Modified Dyspnea Scale (Breathing)

Scale

A   B   C   D   E   F

Severity

0 Nothing at all	1–2 Very slight	3–4 Slight	5–6 Moderate	7–8 Severe	9. Very severe 10. Maximum

Signs & Symptoms of Left Heart Failure

- Fatigue, dyspnea, or shortness of breath w/mild exercise
- Unable to lie flat due to dyspnea or shortness of breath (orthopnea)
- Getting up suddenly at night to breathe (PND)
- Decreased ejection fraction (<40%)
- Interstitial or pulmonary edema on chest x-ray
- Bibasilar crackles or rales
- Weight gain of 2–3 lb overnight is a sign of decompensation

Signs & Symptoms of Right Heart Failure

- Fatigue, dyspnea, or shortness of breath w/mild exercise
- Edema in bilateral LEs, bilateral hands, swollen abdomen, liver congestion
- JVD (jugular venous distention)
- Cyanosis and/or decreased PaO_2 or SpO_2

Signs & Symptoms of Abdominal Aneurysm

- Chest pain w/palpable pulsating mass (abdomen)
- Abdominal heart beat felt when lying down
- Dull ache in mid-abdominal left flank or low back pain
- Groin and/or leg pain
- Weakness or transient paralysis of legs

Signs & Symptoms of Arterial Disease

- Intermittent claudication
- Burning, ischemic pain at rest
- Resting pain increased w/elevating extremity; relieved w/dangling foot over side of bed or chair
- Poor nail and hair growth
- Poor circulation/healing and possible ulceration and gangrene in most distal aspects of lower extremities

Signs & Symptoms of Orthostatic Hypotension

- Drop in systolic BP >10 mm Hg with increase in HR and symptoms
- Lightheadedness or dizziness with upright position

- Syncope or fainting upon assuming upright position
- Mental or visual blurring
- Weakness/wobbly legs upon assuming stand

Signs & Symptoms of Raynaud Disease

Symptoms occur w/exposure to cold or strong emotion.
- Cyanosis or blueness of digits
- Cold, numbness, and pain of digits
- Intense redness of digits

Exercise Assessments

Gait Speed Assessment 6 M or 20 M

Used for functional assessment
Convert distance walked (4 m or 10 m) divided by time to walk distance
and convert to meters/1 second
- Either 20-m distance w/5-m acceleration and deceleration and 10-m
  timed walk distance

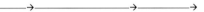

5-m acceleration   10-m timed walk   5-m deceleration
- OR
- 6-m and 1-m acceleration and deceleration and 4-m timed walk
  distance

Walking Speed
[meter per second (m/s)]

0	0.2	0.4	0.6	0.8	1	1.2	1.4
	Dependent in ADLs and IADLs					Independent in ADLs	
	More likely to be hospitalized					Less likely to be hospitalized	
			Need intervention to reduce falls risk			Less likely to have adverse event	
D/C to SNF	D/C to home more likely						
	Household walker		Limited community ambulator		Community ambulator		Cross street and normal WS

0 mph	0.4 mph	0.9 mph	1.3 mph	1.8 mph	2.2 mph	2.7 mph	3.1 mph
10 meter walk time	50 sec	25 sec	16.7 sec	12.5 sec	10 sec	8.3 sec	7.1 sec
10 foot walk time	15.2 sec	7.6 sec	5 sec	3.8 sec	3 sec	2.5 sec	2.2 sec

Six-Minute Walk Test

Timed walk test to measure patient/client exercise endurance by observing distance covered in 6 min

- Use a specific measured path (optimal length: 100 ft); mark the walking surface at 10-ft intervals; chair avail every 50 ft
- Patient/client walks at regular pace while therapist monitors SpO_2 & level of dyspnea for 6 min
- Patient/client carries or wheels own O_2 & may rest when needed, but timing continues during rests
- Record distance, SpO_2, level of dyspnea, and number of rests
- Equipment: Stopwatch, 6-min walk documentation form, steth & sphygmomanometer, pulse oximetry, and, if needed, supplemental O_2 and/or telemetry

Shuttle Walk Test

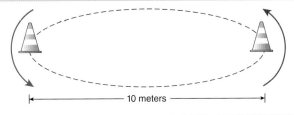

Level	Speed m/s		Distance Ambulated at the End of Each Level (m)
1	0.50	3	30
2	0.67	4	70
3	0.84	5	120
4	1.01	6	180
5	1.18	7	250
6	1.35	8	330
7	1.52	9	420
8	1.69	10	520
9	1.86	11	630
10	2.03	12	750
11	2.20	13	880
12	2.37	14	1000

Treadmill Tests: Most Common Protocols

Bruce Test*		
Speed	**Grade**	**Time**
1.7 mph	10%	3 min
2.5 mph	12%	3 min
3.4 mph	14%	3 min
4.2 mph	16%	3 min
5.0 mph	18%	3 min

*Used most often in hospitals for diagnostic purposes

Balke Test
■ Most often used for athletes
■ Start: 3.3 mph, 0%, grade ↑ 1% every min

Harbor/Ramp Test
Start walking at comfortable speed, ↑ grade each minute depending on fitness level

Naughton Protocol				
Stages	**Speed**	**Grade**	**Time**	**METs**
0	1 mph	0%	2 min	1.6 METs*
I	2 mph	0%	2 min	2 METs*
II	2 mph	3.5%	2 min	3 METs*
III	2 mph	7%	2 min	4 METs*
IV	2 mph	10.5%	2 min	5 METs*
V	2 mph	14%	2 min	6 METs*
VI	2 mph	17.5%	2 min	7 METs

*METs are metabolic equivalent of task: 1 MET = oxygen consumption for individual sitting at rest or 3.5 ml O_2/kg/min. All other METs are multiples of 1 MET and are an estimate of oxygen cost of tasks.

Abnormal Signs and Symptoms

S/S	Abnormal Responses
Blood pressure	• Abnormally high BP rise: systolic >240 mm Hg • Diastolic >110 mm Hg • Exercise hypotension (>10 mm Hg; systolic ↓ w/↑ activity)
ABN HR response	• Rapid ↑ from rest in relation to activity • Failure to ↑ w/↑ activity
Symptoms of intolerance	• ↓ w/↑ activity (often indicates arrhythmia) • Significant ↑ in angina • Excessive dyspnea • Excessive fatigue • Mental confusion or dizziness • Leg claudication
Signs	• Excessive fatigue • Mental confusion or dizziness • Leg claudication • Cold sweat • Ataxia • New heart murmur • Pallor • Auscultation of pulmonary rales • Onset of significant third heart sound (S_3) • Drop in SpO_2
ECG	• Serious arrhythmias (multifocal PVCs, couplets, triplets, etc) • Second- or third-degree AV block • Acute ST changes

Sternal Precautions Algorithm

Risk of sternal complications

Number of primary & secondary risk factors
Sternal instability scale score
Patient characteristics/clinical profile

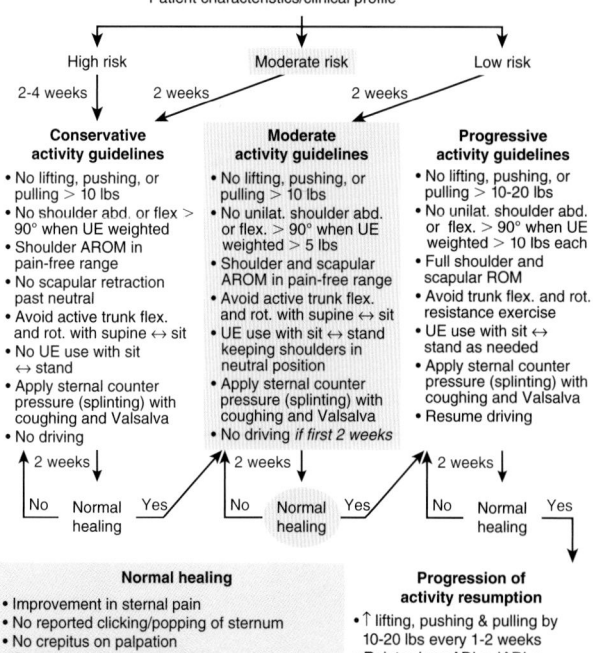

High risk

2-4 weeks

Moderate risk

2 weeks

Low risk

2 weeks

Conservative activity guidelines

- No lifting, pushing, or pulling > 10 lbs
- No shoulder abd. or flex > 90° when UE weighted
- Shoulder AROM in pain-free range
- No scapular retraction past neutral
- Avoid active trunk flex. and rot. with supine ↔ sit
- No UE use with sit ↔ stand
- Apply sternal counter pressure (splinting) with coughing and Valsalva
- No driving

Moderate activity guidelines

- No lifting, pushing, or pulling > 10 lbs
- No unilat. shoulder abd. or flex. > 90° when UE weighted > 5 lbs
- Shoulder and scapular AROM in pain-free range
- Avoid active trunk flex. and rot. with supine ↔ sit
- UE use with sit ↔ stand keeping shoulders in neutral position
- Apply sternal counter pressure (splinting) with coughing and Valsalva
- No driving *if first 2 weeks*

Progressive activity guidelines

- No lifting, pushing, or pulling > 10-20 lbs
- No unilat. shoulder abd. or flex. > 90° when UE weighted > 10 lbs each
- Full shoulder and scapular ROM
- Avoid trunk flex. and rot. resistance exercise
- UE use with sit ↔ stand as needed
- Apply sternal counter pressure (splinting) with coughing and Valsalva
- Resume driving

↑ 2 weeks ↓

No   Normal healing   Yes

2 weeks

No   Normal healing   Yes

2 weeks

No   Normal healing   Yes

Normal healing

- Improvement in sternal pain
- No reported clicking/popping of sternum
- No crepitus on palpation
- Complete cutaneous healing
- No signs or symptoms of local or systemic infection

Progression of activity resumption

- ↑ lifting, pushing & pulling by 10-20 lbs every 1-2 weeks
- Reintroduce ADLs, IADLs, occupational & recreational tasks

Cardiopulmonary Diagnostics

Diagnostic Tests	Indications	Info Gathered From Tests	Precautions & Notes
CXR	Eval of anatomic abnormalities & pathological process in lungs & chest wall	Lung size, heart size Integrity of ribs, sternum, clavicles, vascular markings Chronic vs. acute Δ Lung fields: size, presence of fluid/secretions, hyper/ hypoinflation Presence of pleural fluid	AP films are often taken while patient/ client is in bed; therefore patient/clients often have hypo-inflation due to a poor effort
ECG	Eval of chest pain to determine if acute injury; eval of hypertrophy or old infarction (injury); eval of heart rhythm	Heart rhythm Old MI Vent/atrial hypertrophy Acute ischemia, injury, infarction conduction defects	Cannot predict ischemia or infarction; stress test used to predict
Echocardiogram	Eval of valve function &/or chamber sizes	Integrity, function of valves Chamber size, eval of pericardial sac	Noninvasive
Holter monitoring	Eval of heart rhythm; eval of syncope	24-hour recording of rhythm of heart	Noninvasive

Continued

Diagnostic Tests	Indications	Info Gathered From Tests	Precautions & Notes
CT, spiral CT, or MRI	ABN CXR showing nodule or mass	Enhanced pictures for interpretation of nodules or masses Spiral CT is gold standard for identifying pulmonary embolism	Noninvasive but CT does produce radiation exposure
Stress testing, exercise stress, nuclear imaging w/exercise stress, 2D/3D echo w/exercise, pharmacological stress (adenosine, dobut)	Determine aerobic capacity Assess whether myocardial O_2 supply meets demand (assess for chest pain/ coronary artery disease/ ischemia)	Max VO_2, HR, BP response to activity, assessment of chest pain Assess ischemia Presence/absence of arrhythmias Limitation to exercise	Women have ↑ rates of false-positive & false-negative tests Need to have additional imaging w/ stress testing (thallium, 2D/3D echo)
Coronary catheterization	Chest pain, infarction	Blood flow through & integrity of coronary arteries Pressure changes across valves Estimated ejection fraction	Allergy to dye if patient/client has allergy to shellfish or iodine 24 hours of bedrest post cath through femoral artery

Cardiopulmonary Diagnostics—cont'd

Diagnostic Tests	Indications	Info Gathered From Tests	Precautions & Notes
V/Q scans	Rule out pulmonary emboli, especially in DVT	Gas distribution in lungs Regional ventilation matching of alveolar vent & pulm perfusion	Reliability of test is related to technician and interpretation
Bronchoscopy	Obtain sputum sample for infection, malignancy; to clear viscous secretions not mobilized by patient/client	Direct visualization of inaccessible areas of bronchial tree	May induce bronchospasm
PFT	Classification of disease: obstructive vs. restrictive; assess severity of disease or severity of acute illness	Integrity of airways Function of respiratory musculature Condition of lung tissues	Patient must have enough strength/ endurance to produce a good effort

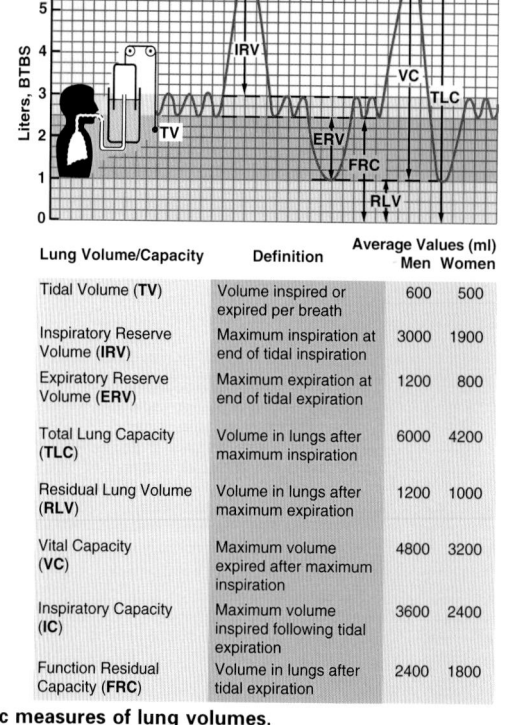

Lung Volume/Capacity	Definition	Average Values (ml)	
		Men	Women
Tidal Volume (**TV**)	Volume inspired or expired per breath	600	500
Inspiratory Reserve Volume (**IRV**)	Maximum inspiration at end of tidal inspiration	3000	1900
Expiratory Reserve Volume (**ERV**)	Maximum expiration at end of tidal expiration	1200	800
Total Lung Capacity (**TLC**)	Volume in lungs after maximum inspiration	6000	4200
Residual Lung Volume (**RLV**)	Volume in lungs after maximum expiration	1200	1000
Vital Capacity (**VC**)	Maximum volume expired after maximum inspiration	4800	3200
Inspiratory Capacity (**IC**)	Maximum volume inspired following tidal expiration	3600	2400
Function Residual Capacity (**FRC**)	Volume in lungs after tidal expiration	2400	1800

Static measures of lung volumes.

Redrawn from McArdle WD, Katch FI, Katch VL: Exercise Physiology: Energy, Nutrition, and Human Performance, 4th ed. Williams & Wilkins, Baltimore, 1996.

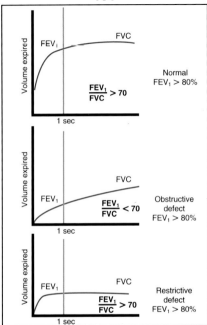

Dynamic lung measurements.

Redrawn from McArdle WD, Katch FI, Katch VL: Exercise Physiology: Energy, Nutrition, and Human Performance, 4th ed. Williams & Wilkins, Baltimore, 1996.

Stages of COPD

Severity	Symptoms	Spirometry	Treatment
Stage I: Mild	Chronic cough; occasional white/clear sputum	FEV_1/FVC <70% FEV_1 ≥80% predicted	Often no treatment required except during respiratory illness. Should be treated with pneumonia and flu vaccines
Stage II: Moderate	Development of dyspnea on exertion (DOE) w/chronic cough and occasional to regular sputum	FEV_1/FVC <70% FEV_1 50% to 79% predicted	Often long-acting bronchodilator prescribed Rehabilitation should be considered
Stage III: Severe	Repeated exacerbations, DOE, chronic cough & sputum	FEV_1/FVC <70% FEV_1 30% to 49% predicted	Long-acting bronchodilators plus inhaled glucocorticoids especially w/exacerbations; Rehabilitation should be considered
Stage IV: Very Severe	Quality of life impaired, several exacerbations	FEV_1/FVC <70% FEV_1 <30% predicted or <50%, plus chronic respiratory failure or RHF	Treatment of LABA, inhaled glucocorticosteroids & possibly long-term oxygen therapy if chronic hypoxemia

ECG/Arrhythmias

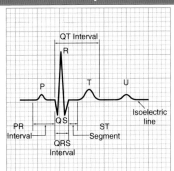

Components of an ECG tracing.

From Jones, SA: ECG Notes, Philadelphia, FA Davis Co., 2005.

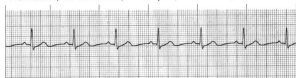

Normal sinus rhythm.

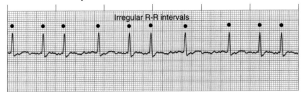

Atrial fibrillation; irregular/irregular heart rhythm, no discernible P waves.

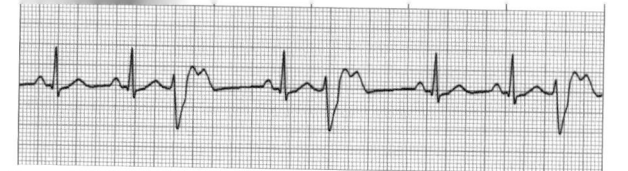

Premature ventricular contraction: uniform (same form) (wide, bizarre QRS, w/o P wave before).

From Jones SA: ECG Notes, Philadelphia, F.A. Davis Co., 2005.

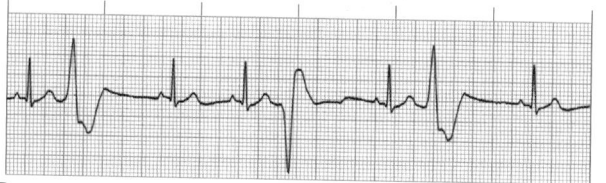

Premature ventricular contraction: multiform (different forms) (wide, bizarre QRS, w/o P wave before, & aberrant beats look different).

From Jones SA: ECG Notes, Philadelphia, F.A. Davis Co., 2005.

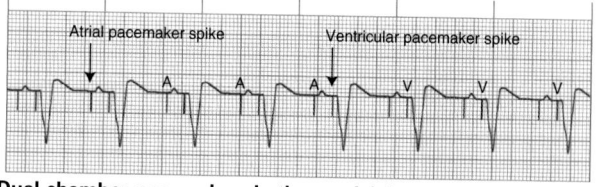

Dual-chamber pacemaker rhythm: atrial & ventricular vertical line before P wave, and/or QRS indicates pacemaker firing.

From Jones SA: ECG Notes, Philadelphia, F.A. Davis Co., 2005.

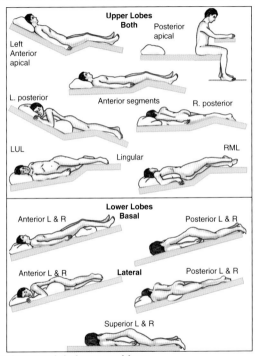

Typical postural drainage positions.

Redrawn from White, GC: Basic Clinical Competencies for Respiratory Care: An Integrated Approach. Albany, NY, Delmar Publishers, 1988.

Exercise Prescription for Aerobic Exercise

Mode	Est ↑ VO$_2$ max w/exercise using large muscle groups over long time: walk, run, bike, etc
Intensity	Most commonly used: HR or RPE (see next table)
Frequency	Optimal: 3–5x/wk unless duration is <10–15 min; may work 7x/wk if very poor exercise tolerance
Duration	Optimal: 20–30 min >30 min for wt loss programs <20 min for poor exercise tolerance: perform multiple short bouts

Heart Rate Methods for Determining Intensity

% HR max	Target HR (THR) should be 55%–75% of HR max
HR Reserve	THR = (HR max – HR rest) × (0.60–0.80) + HR rest
Deconditioned	Use lower % (40–60) or (0.40–0.60)

Caloric Cost of Exercise Estimation

$$(METs × 3.5 × body\ wt\ in\ kg)/200 = kcal/min$$
$$1\ MET = 3.5\ mL\ O_2/kg/min$$

Leisure Activities in METs

Activity	Mean	Range
Bowling	2.5	2–4
Conditioning exercise		3–8+
Dancing (aerobic)		6–9
Golf (cart use)		2–3
Running (12-min mile)	8.7	
Running (9-min mile)	11.2	
Skiing (downhill)		5–8

Leisure Activities in METs—cont'd

Activity	Mean	Range
Soccer		5–12+
Tennis	6.5	4–9+

Indications for Referral

Indications for Referral	Suggested Referral Source
Elevated lipids (LDL, total chol, triglyc)	Dietitian, physician for lipid-lowering meds
Elevated blood glucose	Physician to evaluate for diabetes (possibly an endocrinologist), dietitian
↑ BMI	Dietitian, exercise program
Low albumin/prealbumin	Dietitian
ABN thyroid profile	Physician (possibly an endocrinologist)
Elevated BP	Physician for ↑ BP, meds, exercise program, dietitian
Continues to smoke	Smoking cessation program
Demonstrates anger/hostility easily	Psychologist/behavior specialist
Demonstrates s/s of depression	Psychologist/behavior specialist, physician for meds
Sedentary lifestyle	Exercise program
Elevated BMI or wt	Dietitian, exercise program

Special Considerations/Populations

Transplants (Heart & Lung)

Complications w/Heart & Lung Transplants

Immunosuppressive Med Side Effects
- Renal dysfunction
- Hypertension

- Mood swings
- Skeletal muscle atrophy
- Osteoporosis
- ABN blood lipid profile

Acute Rejection
- Risk for opportunistic infections & malignancy
- Accelerated graft coronary artery disease in heart transplant patient/ clients

Signs & Symptoms of Acute Rejection
- Low-grade fever
- ↑ in resting blood pressure
- Hypotension w/activities
- Myalgias
- Fatigue
- ↓ exercise tolerance

Ventricular Arrhythmias

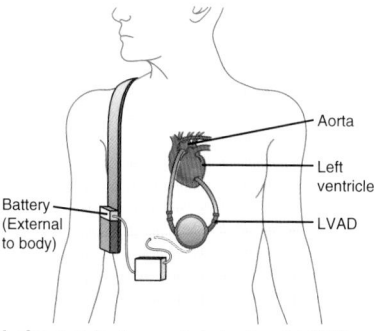

Left ventricular assist device (LVAD).

Considerations for exercise testing & training in patient/clients w/LVAD:

- Type of LVAD:
  - Location of externalized drive line makes cycling & climbing stairs difficult
  - HR response (palpated or from ECG) normal

- BP response variable due to fluid volume adjustment
- Consider skeletal muscle impairment if patient/client experienced long-standing CHF prior to LVAD

Responses to Activity in Cardiac Transplant Patient/Clients

Physiological Variables	Responses in Cardiac Transplant Patient/Clients
Rest HR	Elevated (>90 bpm)
Rest BP	Mildly elevated unless affected by meds
HR response to increasing activity	No $\triangle$ first 5–10 min, followed by gradual rise w/activity
Peak HR	Slightly lower than normal (approx 150 bpm); often achieved during first few min of recovery
BP response to increasing activity	NL; peak BP lower than expected
Systemic vascular resistance	Generally elevated
Pulmonary vascular pressures	Generally elevated
Left vent systolic function (EF)	NL range at rest & w/exercise
Diastolic function (EDV)	Impaired: results in below normal $\uparrow$ in SV w/exercise
Skeletal muscle abnormalities	Greater reliance on anaerobic metabolic energy production
Ventilation	Efficiency is below normal $\uparrow$ VE/VCO$_2$: $\uparrow$ sense of SOB $\downarrow$ rise in tidal volume w/exercise Diffusion impairment
Arterial-mixed venous O$_2$ content (a-vO$_2$ diff)	NL at rest, impaired w/exercise

Patient/Clients w/Pacemakers, ICDs, & IABP

Invasive Monitoring or Device	Implications for Rehab Professionals
Pacemakers Fixed rate (FR) Demand (D) A-V sequential	Identify type of pacemaker FR: HR will not ↑ w/activity; will make heart contract at SET HR D: HR will ↑ w/activity Pacemaker initiates vent contraction when HR drops below a set rate A-V: Most common pacemaker; atria stimulated to depolarize, then ventricles Left UE ROM above shoulder restricted for 24–72 hr after implant
ICD	Corrects life-threatening arrhythmias Used in high risk for sudden death pop Left UE ROM above shoulder restricted for 24–72 hr after implant
IABP	Used to ↑ diastolic BP & ↑ coronary blood flow. Use: hemodynamically unstable patient/client. Hip flexion kept <70°. OOB contraind. Only ROM & bed mobility

Evaluation Notes for Practice Pattern

Patterns	Included Diagnoses	Prognosis
6A: Primary prevention & risk reduction for CV/pulmonary disorders	Diabetes, obesity, hypertension, sedentary lifestyle, smoking, hypercholesterolemia, hyperlipidemia	Patient/client will ↓ risk for CV/pulmonary disorders w/therapeutic exercise, aerobic conditioning, functional training, & lifestyle modification
6B: Impaired aerobic cap/endur associated w/deconditioning	AIDS, cancer, CV disorders, chronic systems failure, inactivity, multisystem impairments, musculoskeletal disorders, neuromuscular disorders, pulmonary disorders	In 6–12 wk, patient/client will demonstrate optimal aerobic cap/endur & >established level of function in home, work, community, & leisure environs

Evaluation Notes for Practice Pattern—cont'd

Patterns	Included Diagnoses	Prognosis
6C: Impaired ventilation, resp/ gas exchange, & aerobic cap/ endur associated w/airway clearance dysfunction	Acute lung disorders, acute/chronic O_2 dependency, bone marrow/stem cell transplants, cardiothoracic surgery, Δ in baseline breath sounds, Δ in baseline CXR, COPD, frequent/ recurring pulmonary infection, solid-organ transplants, tracheostomy or microtracheostomy	In 12–16 wk, patient/client will demonstrate optimal vent, resp. and/or gas exchange, & aerobic cap/endur & >est level of function in home, work, community, & leisure environs within the context of the impairment
6D: Impaired aerobic cap/endur associated w/CV pump dysfunction or failure	Angioplasty/atherectomy, AV block, cardiogenic shock, cardiomyopathy, cardiothoracic surgery, complex vent arrhythmia, complicated myocardial infarction (failure), uncomplicated myocardial infarction (dysfunction), congenital cardiac abnormalities, coronary artery disease, ↓ ejection fraction (<50%), diabetes, exercise-induced myocardial ischemia, hypertensive heart disease, nonmalignant arrhythmias, valvular heart disease	In 6–12 wk, patient/client w/CV **pump dysfunction** will show opt aerobic cap/endur & >est level of function in home, work, community, & leisure environs w/in context of impairment, functional limits, & disabilities In 8–16 wk, patient/client w/CV **pump failure** will show optimal aerobic cap/endur (etc)

Evaluation Notes for Practice Pattern—cont'd

Patterns	Included Diagnoses	Prognosis
6E: Impaired ventilation & resp/gas exchange associated w/ ventilatory pump dysfunction or failure	Elevated diaphragm + volume loss on CXR, neuromuscular disorders, partial/complete diaphragmatic paralysis, poliomyelitis, pulmonary fibrosis, restrictive lung disease, severe kyphoscoliosis, spinal/ cerebral neoplasm, spinal cord injury	In 3–6 wk, patient/client w/**vent pump dysfunction or reversible vent pump failure will show opt** independence w/vent & resp/ gas exchange & < level of function in home, work, community, & leisure environs, within context of impairment, functional limits, & disabilities In 9–10 wk, patient/client w/**prolonged, severe, or chronic vent pump failure will demonstrate optimal** independence w/vent & resp/ gas exchange & (etc)
6F: Impaired vent & resp/gas exchange associated w/ respiratory failure	ABN CXR, acute neuromuscular dysfunction, ARDS, ABN alveolar to arterial oxygen tension differences, asthma, cardiothoracic surgery, COPD, inability to maintain O_2 tension w/supplemental O_2, multisystem failure, pneumonia, pre/post lung transplant or rejection, rapid rise in arterial CO_2 at rest or w/activity, sepsis, thoracic or multisystem trauma	Within 72 hr, patient/client w/**acute reversible resp failure will demonstrate optimal** independence w/vent & resp/ gas exchange & > established level of function in home, work, community, & leisure environs Within 3 wk, patient/client w/**prolonged resp failure will demonstrate optimal indep** w/vent, (etc) In 4–6 wk, patient/client w/**severe or chronic resp failure will demonstrate optimal indep** w/vent, (etc)

Evaluation Notes for Practice Pattern—cont'd

Patterns	Included Diagnoses	Prognosis
6G: Impaired vent, resp/gas exchange, & aerobic cap/ endur associated w/resp failure in the neonate	ABN thoracic surgeries, apnea & bradycardia, bronchopulmonary dysphasia, congenital anomalies, hyaline membrane disease, meconium aspiration syndrome, neurovascular disorders, pneumonia, rapid desaturation w/ movement or crying	In 6–12 mo, patient/client will demonstrate optimal vent, resp/ gas exchange, & aerobic cap/ endur & the > est level of age-appropriate function
6H: Impaired circulation & anthropometric dimensions associated w/ lymphatic system disorders	AIDS, cellulitis, filariasis, infection/sepsis, lymphedema, post-radiation, reconstructive surgery, reflex sympathetic dystrophy, status post lymph node dissection, trauma	Within 1–8 wk, patient/client w/**mild lymphedema** (<3 cm differential between affected limb & unaffected limb) will demonstrate optimal circ & anthrop dimensions & > established level of function in home, work, community, & leisure environs within context of the impairment, functional limits, & disabilities Within 1–8 wk, patient/client w/**moderate lymphedema** (3–5 cm differential) will demonstrate opt circ, etc Within 8 wk, patient/client w/**severe lymphedema** (5 plus cm differential) will demonstrate optimal circ, etc

HAPTA: Guide to Physical Therapist Practice, 2nd ed. Physical Therapy (2001) 81(9), 744.

Assessment of the Lymphatic System

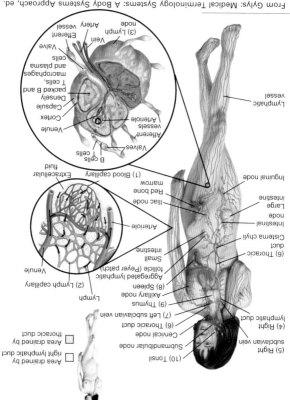

☐ Area drained by right lymphatic duct
☐ Area drained by thoracic duct

Submandibular node
Cervical node
(7) Left subclavian vein
(6) Thoracic duct
(10) Tonsil
(9) Thymus
Axillary node
(8) Spleen
Aggregated lymphatic follicle (Peyer patch)
Small intestine
Cisterna chyli
(6) Thoracic duct
Intestinal node
Large intestine
Inguinal node
Lymphatic vessel

Right subclavian vein (5)
(4) Right lymphatic duct

Iliac node
Red bone marrow
(1) Blood capillary

Arteriole
(2) Lymph capillary
Lymph
Venule
Extracellular fluid

(3) Lymph node
Artery
Efferent vessel
Vein
Valve
Densely packed B and T cells, macrophages and plasma cells
Capsule
Cortex
Venule
Arteriole
Afferent vessels
Valves
B cells   T cells

From Gylys: Medical Terminology Systems: A Body Systems Approach, ed. 5. Philadelphia, F.A. Davis, 2003, p 255.

114

ICD 10 Codes for Neurological Impairments

G00-G99 Diseases of the Nervous System

G00-09	Inflammatory diseases of the central nervous system
G10-13	Systemic atrophies primarily affecting the central nervous system
G20-26	Extrapyramidal and movement disorders
G30-32	Other degenerative diseases of the nervous system
G35-37	Demyelinating diseases of the central nervous system
G40-47	Episodic and paroxysmal disorders
G50-59	Nerve, nerve root, and plexus disorders
G60-64	Polyneuropathies and other disorders of the peripheral nervous system
G70-73	Diseases of myoneural junction and muscle
G80-83	Cerebral palsy and other paralytic syndromes
G90-99	Other disorders of the nervous system

R25-R29 Symptoms and Signs Involving the Nervous and Musculoskeletal Systems

R25	Abnormal involuntary movements
R26	Abnormalities of gait and mobility
R27	Other lack of coordination
R29	Other symptoms and signs involving the nervous and musculoskeletal systems

R40-R46 Symptoms and Signs Involving Cognition, Perception, Emotional State, and Behavior

R40	Somnolence, stupor, and coma
R41	Other symptoms and signs involving cognitive functions and awareness
R42	Dizziness and giddiness
R43	Disturbances of smell and taste
R44	Other symptoms and signs involving general sensations and taste
R45	Symptoms and signs involving emotional state
R46	Symptoms and signs involving appearance and behavior

S00-S29 Injuries

S00-S09	Injuries to the head
S10-S19	Injuries to the neck
S20-S29	Injuries to the thorax
S30-S39	Injuries to the abdomen, lower back, lumbar spine, and pelvis

V01-V59 Accidents: pedestrian and transport

Quick Screen for Neurological Dysfunction

Motor control assessment: All areas should be checked as ABN vs NL.

NL	ABN	Test
—	—	Cognition
—	—	Communication
—	—	Arousal
—	—	Sensation
—	—	Perception
—	—	Flexibility
—	—	Tone
—	—	Deep tendon reflexes
—	—	Developmental reflexes
—	—	Righting reactions
—	—	Muscle strength
—	—	Movement patterns
—	—	Coordination
—	—	Balance
—	—	Gait
—	—	Functional abilities

Neurological Assessment

Memory Tests

The Mini-Mental Status Examination
The MMS is a quick way to quantify cognitive function and screen for deficiency. It tests orientation, attention, calculation, recall, language, and motor skills. Seat the individual in a quiet, well-lit room. Ask him/her to

From World Health Organization. International Statistical Classification of Diseases, ed. 10. http://apps.who.int/classifications/icd10/browse/2010/en with permission.

listen carefully and to answer each question as accurately as he/she can. Score one point for each correct answer. To score, add the number of correct responses. Max score = 30. Below 20 indicates cognitive impairment.

The Mini-Mental Status Examination

Orientation to Time	Correct	Incorrect
What is today's date?		
What is the month?		
What is the year?		
What is the day of the week today?		
What season is it?		
Total: ___/5		
Orientation to Place		
Whose home is this?		
What room is this?		
What city are we in?		
What county are we in?		
What state are we in?		
Total: ___/5		
Immediate Recall: Ask if you may test his/her memory. Then say, "ball," "flag," "tree" clearly and slowly, about 1 sec for each. After you have said all 3 words, ask him/her to repeat them—the first repetition determines the score (0–3):		
Ball		
Flag		
Tree		
Total: ___/3		

Continued

Orientation to Time	Correct	Incorrect
Attention: A) Ask the individual to begin w/100 and count backward by 7s. Stop after 5 subtractions. Score the correct subtractions.		
93		
86		
79		
72		
65		
Total: ___/5		
B) Ask the individual to spell the word "world" backward. The score is the number of letters in correct position.		
D		
L		
R		
O		
W		
Total ___/5		
Delayed Verbal Recall: Ask the individual to recall the 3 words you previously asked him/her to remember.		
Ball		
Flag		
Tree		
Total: ___/3		
Naming: Show the individual a wristwatch and ask him/her what it is. Repeat for a pencil.		
Watch		
Pencil		
Total ___/2		

The Mini-Mental Status Examination—cont'd

Orientation to Time	Correct	Incorrect
Repetition: Ask the individual to repeat the following: "No if, ands, or buts."		
Total ___/1		
3-Stage Command: Give the individual a plain piece of paper and say, "Take the paper in your hand, fold it in half, and put it on the floor."		
Takes		
Folds		
Puts		
Total: ___/3		
Reading: Hold up the card reading "Close your eyes" so the individual can see it clearly. Ask him/her to read it and do what it says. Score correctly only if the individual actually closes his/her eyes.		
Total ___/1		
Writing: Give the individual a piece of paper and ask him/her to write a sentence. It is to be written spontaneously. It must contain a subject and verb and be sensible.		
Total ___/1		
Copying: Give the individual a piece of paper and ask him/her to copy a design of two intersecting shapes. One point is awarded for correctly copying the shapes. All angles on both figures must be present, and the figures must have one overlapping angle.		
Total ___/1		
Total Score:_____		

From "Mini-mental state." *A practical method for grading the cognitive state of patients for the clinician.* Journal of Psychiatric Research, 12(3): 189–198, 1975. Used by permission.

Mental Status Tests

Elements Tested	Description	Examples of Tests
Level of consciousness	Alert Lethargic Obtunded Stupor Coma	Observation by family
Attention	Ability to focus and remain w/o distraction on a stimulus or task	Ask about medical Hx, recite months backward, recite a list of digits provided
Orientation	Person Place Time	What is your name? Where are you? What day/year is it? Who is the current president?
Language function	Fluency Repetition Comprehension Spontaneous speech Naming and word finding	Questions on personal events, word problems, fam, common interests
Reading & writing	Learning & memory Immediate recall Short- & long-term	Recall of distant news events, math problems Word problems
Cortical & cognitive functions	Fund of knowledge Ability to perform calculations Proverb interpretation Praxia/apraxia Gnosia/agnosia	Calculations Recall of messages Proverbs
Mood & affect	Feelings, emotions, & somatic & autonomic behaviors: determine if appropriate in current situation	Observation
Thought content	Fullness & organization of thinking: (paranoia, disordered thought content)	Stories, personal experiences, & fam Hx questions

Modified Hachinski Scale

This scale is sometimes used by clinicians to assess the probability of avascular dementia.

Item	Score
Abrupt onset	2
Stepwise loss	1
Somatic complaints	1
Emotional incontinence	1
History of hypertension	1
History of stroke	2
Focal neurological symptoms	2
Focal neurological signs	2

Score ≥4 suggests cerebrovascular contribution to dementia.

Diagnostic Criteria for Dementia (DSM-IV Table 8)

Memory impairment: impaired ability to learn new information or to recall old information.
One or more of the following:

■ Aphasia—language disturbance;
■ Apraxia—impaired ability to carry out motor activities despite intact motor function;
■ Agnosia—failure to recognize or identify objects despite intact sensory function;
■ Disturbance in executive functioning-impaired ability to plan, organize, sequence, abstract.
■ The cognitive deficits result in functional impairment (social/occupational).
■ Cognitive deficits do not occur exclusively solely during a delirium.

NOT due to other medical or psychiatric conditions

The Westmead Post Traumatic Amnesia (PTA) Scale

■ Predictors of long-term outcome following head injury.
■ Uses a series of orientation and memory questions to produce a score from 1 to 12.
■ When consistently achieves a score of 12 over a period of time, patient/client is considered to have emerged from PTA.

Questions

How old are you?
What is your date of birth?
What month are we in?
What time of day is it? (Morning, Afternoon or Night)
What day of the week is it?
What year are we in?
What is the name of this place?
Who do you have to remember? (Show set of 3 photos.)
What is their name?
What were the 3 pictures that you had to remember?
Score is from 1 to 12. One point for each question, 3 points for last question on pictures. Assessment should be done regularly and record total correct/12 and identify questions that were incorrectly answered until person gets all 12 correct; then define length of time in days/weeks.

Traumatic Brain Injury (TBI) Severity Using PTA Scale* Alone	
Severity	**Length of Time Until a Score of 12 Achieved**
Very mild	<5 min
Mild	5–60 min
Moderate	1–24 h
Severe	1–7 d
Very severe	1–4 wk
Extremely severe	>4 wk

*PTA scale is considered to be best measure of head trauma severity; PTA duration is linked to likelihood of having behavioral problems with TBI.

van der Naalt J (2001). "Prediction of outcome in mild to moderate head injury: A review". *Journal of Clinical and Experimental Neuropsychology* **23** (6): 837–851.

Galveston Orientation and Amnesia Test (GOAT)

Questions	Scoring (score only errors)
What is your name?	-2 (must give first and last name)
When were you born?	-4 (must give day, month, year)
Where do you live?	-4 (town is sufficient)
Where are you now? City? Building?	-5 (must give actual town) -5 (actual name necessary)
When were you admitted to this hospital?	-5 (date)
How did you get here?	-5 (mode of transport)
What is the first event you can remember after the injury?	-5 (any plausible event is sufficient)
Can you give some detail?	-5 (must give relevant detail
Can you describe the last event you can recall before the accident?	-5 (any plausible event)
What time is it now?	-5 (-1 for each ½ hour error)
What day of the week is it?	-3 (-1 for each day error)
What day of the month is it? (What is the date?)	-5 (-1 for each day error)
What is the month?	-15 (-5 for each month error)
What is the year?	-30 (-10 for each year error)
Total Error	
Total actual score = 100 – total error	76–100 = Normal 66–75 = borderline <66 impaired

Instructions: *Can be administered daily.*
Levin HS, O'Donnell VM, Grossman RG. The Galveston Orientation and Amnesia Test. A practical scale to assess cognition after head injury. *J Nerv Ment Dis.* 1979 Nov;167(11):675–84.

Glasgow Coma Scale

Eyes	Verbal	Motor	Points
No opening of eyes	No sounds	No movements	1
Eyes open in response to painful stimuli	Incomprehensible sounds	Responds to painful stimuli w/extension posture (decerebrate)	2
Eyes open in response to voice	Utters inappropriate words	Responds to painful stimuli w/flexion posture (decorticate)	3
Opens eyes spontaneously	Confused/disoriented	Flexion/withdrawal to painful stimuli	4
	Oriented, converses normally	Localizes painful stimuli	5
		Obeys commands	6

The three values separately as well as their sum are considered.
The lowest possible GCS (sum) is 3 = deep coma or death. Highest is 15 = fully awake.
Brain injury is defined as Severe ≤8; Moderate 9–12; Minor ≥13.

Levels of TBI Severity

	GCS	PTA	LOC
Mild	13–15	<1 h	<30 min
Moderate	9–12	30 min–24 h	1–24 h
Severe	3–8	>1 d	>24 h

GCS = Glasgow Coma Scale; PTA = post traumatic amnesia scale; LOC = loss of consciousness

Rancho Los Amigos Cognitive Function Scale

Score	Scale Description
X	Purposeful & appropriate: handles multiple tasks simultaneously in all environs/may require breaks. Independently initiates assistive memory devices.
IX	Purposeful & appropriate: independently shifts back & forth between tasks, completes accurately for 2 h Uses assistive memory devices
VIII	Purposeful & appropriate: recalls past & recent events & aware of environment Shows carryover for new learning
VII	Automatic—appropriate: appears appropriately & oriented in hospital & home settings/robot-like
VI	Confused—appropriate: depends on external input or direction/follows simple directions
V	Confused—inappropriate: responds to simple commands consistently/responses not appropriate w/↑ complexity & lack of external structure
IV	Confused/agitated: heightened state of activity/bizarre behavior/nonpurposeful
III	Localized response: reacts specifically but inconsistently to stimuli
II	Generalized response: reacts inconsistently & nonpurposefully to stimuli in nonspecific way
I	No response

Common Causes of Unconsciousness

Condition	Manifestation
Acute alcoholism	Stuporous; responds to noxious stimuli; alcoholic breath; eyes moderately dilated; equal reactive pupils; respirations deep and noisy; blood alcohol >200 mg/dL
Cranial trauma	Often local evidence or Hx of injury; pupils unequal & sluggish or inactive; pulse variable; BP variable; reflexes altered; may have incontinence & paralysis; CT reveals intracranial hemorrhage or fracture
Stroke: ischemia or hemorrhage	Usually Hx of CVD or hypertension; sudden onset w/asymmetry; pupils unequal & inactive; focal neurological signs; hemiplegia
Epilepsy	Sudden convulsive onset; may have incontinence; pupils reactive; tongue bitten or scarred
Diabetic acidosis	Onset gradual; skin dry; face flushed; fruity breath odor; hyperventilation, ketonuria, hyperglycemia, metabolic acidosis in blood
Hypoglycemia	Onset may be acute w/convulsions: preceded by lightheadedness, sweating, nausea, cold/clammy skin, palpitations, headache, hunger. Hypothermia, pupils reactive, deep reflexes exaggerated, + Babinski sign
Syncope	Onset sudden, assoc w/emotional crisis or heart block; coma seldom deep or prolonged; pallor; slow pulse, later rapid & weak. Awakens promptly when supine
Drugs	Cause of 70% of acute coma w/unknown cause

Sensory Testing

Pain: Sharp/Dull
↓ when crossed spinothalamic tract cut (eg, for chronic pain)
Method: Use pin & dull object (use sharp & dull parts of same pin): ask, "Without looking, tell me if object is sharp or dull"

Temperature
Identifies dysfunction in anterolateral pathways
Method: Use hot & cold tap water in tube: "Tell me if object feels warm or cold"

Light Touch
↓: look for anatomic pattern for nerve injury; ABN in multiple nerve & root areas: brain/brainstem lesion
↓ in all extremities: peripheral polyneuropathy
+ loss of motor: spinal cord injury
Method: Dab cotton ball on skin; ask when and where touched

Position Sense
↓: dysfunction of joint or muscle receptors, disease in large myelinated primary afferents, or sensory processing center dysfunction
Method: Passive joint (fingers, toes, wrist, or ankle) displacement

Vibration
↓: peripheral nerve disease affecting large fibers (demyelinated neuropathy) or in central demyelination; shows functional recovery of demyelinated nerve fibers
Method: After tapping tuning fork to set it, apply fork handle to bony prominences & nails

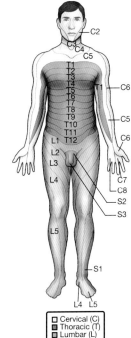

Dermatones.

□ Cervical (C)
■ Thoracic (T)
□ Lumbar (L)
■ Sacral (S)

Stereognosis

↓ w/lesion of multiple ascending pathways or parietal lobe

Method: Patient/client asked to identify common objects placed in hand

Two-Point Discrimination

Crude measure of discriminative sensation

Determines spatial localization

Method: Compass w/blunted tips applied w/↓ distances between tips until one tip reported

Bilateral Simultaneous Stimulation

Parietal lobe disease: feel stimulus on one side only

Method: With subject's eyes closed, lightly touch one side, then other side of body; patient/client determines which side & where

Graphesthesis

↓ w/damage to dorsal columns, medial lemniscus, ventral post thalamus, or parietal lobe

Method: Tracing letters or numbers w/finger on palmar surface of hand

Classification of Clinical Tests of Sensory Function

Functional System	Clinical Tests
Anterolateral systems	Pin prick, thermal sense, deep pain
Dorsal column: medial lemniscus	Light touch, vibratory sense Position sense
Cortical sensory function	Traced figure identification Object identification, double simultaneous stimulation

Referred Pain Patterns: Pain Referred From Viscera

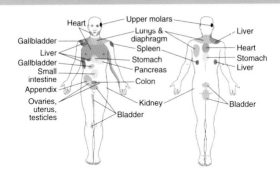

Cranial and Peripheral Nerve Integrity

Cranial Nerves: Functional Components

Number (Name)	Components	Function
I (Olfactory)	Afferent	Smell
II (Optic)	Afferent	Vision
III (Oculomotor)	Efferent (som)	Elevates eyelid, turns eye up, down, in
	Vis	Constricts pupil, accommodates lens
IV (Trochlear)	Efferent	Turns adducted eye down, causes eye twisting
V (Trigeminal)	Mixed, Afferent	Sensation from face, cornea, & anterior tongue
	Efferent	Mastication muscles, dampens sound

Continued

Number (Name)	Components	Function
VI (Abducens)	Efferent	Turns eye out
VII (Facial)	Mixed, Afferent	Taste from anterior tongue
	Efferent (som)	Facial expression muscles Dampens sound
	Efferent (vis)	Tears/salivation
VIII (Vestibulocochlear)	Afferent	Balance (inner ear) Hearing
IX (Glossopharyngeal)	Mixed, Afferent	Taste from posterior tongue Sensation from post-tongue, oropharynx
	Efferent	Salivation (parotid gland)
X (Vagus)	Mixed, Afferent	Thoracic & abdominal viscera
	Efferent	Larynx & pharynx muscles Decreases heart rate Increases GI motility
XI (Spinal Accessory)	Efferent	Head movements Sternocleidomastoid & trapezius
XII (Hypoglossal)	Efferent	Tongue movements & shape

Resisted Muscle Tests for Peripheral Nerve Integrity

Spinal Region Evaluated	Resisted Test for Dysfunction
C1	Cervical rotation force applied
C2, 3, 4	Shoulder elevation resisted
C5	Shoulder abduction resisted
C6	Elbow flexion at 90° resisted Wrist extension resisted
C7	Elbows flexed to 45°, elbow extension resisted Wrist flexion resisted
C8	Thumb extension resisted
T1	Fingers held in abduction resisted
L1, 2	Resisted hip flexion
L3, 4	Resisted dorsiflexion
L5	Great toe extension resisted
S1	Toe walk: 10–20 toe raises
S1, 2	Resisted knee flexion

If painful or painful and weak: muscular pathology.
If painless and weak: neurological disorder.

Physical Rehabilitation: Assess

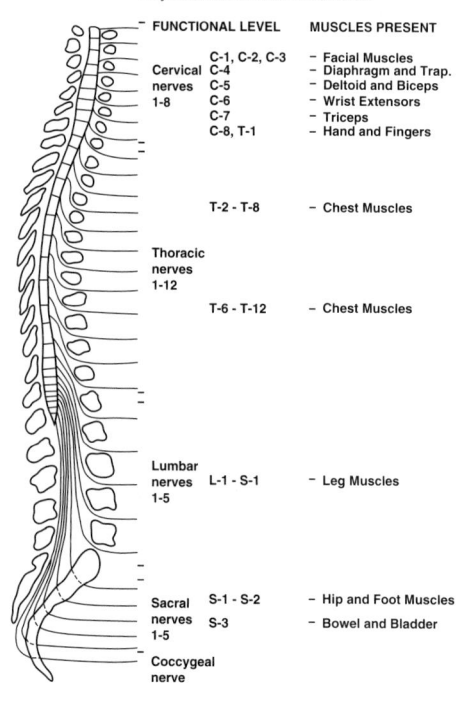

FUNCTIONAL LEVEL		MUSCLES PRESENT
Cervical nerves 1-8	C-1, C-2, C-3	– Facial Muscles
	C-4	– Diaphragm and Trap.
	C-5	– Deltoid and Biceps
	C-6	– Wrist Extensors
	C-7	– Triceps
	C-8, T-1	– Hand and Fingers
	T-2 - T-8	– Chest Muscles
Thoracic nerves 1-12	T-6 - T-12	– Chest Muscles
Lumbar nerves 1-5	L-1 - S-1	– Leg Muscles
Sacral nerves 1-5	S-1 - S-2	– Hip and Foot Muscles
	S-3	– Bowel and Bladder
Coccygeal nerve		

Reflex Integrity

Grading Scale for Muscle Stretch Reflexes

Grade	Evaluation	Response Characteristics
0	Absent	No muscle contraction w/reinforcement (palpable or visible)
1+	Hyporeflexic	Slight or slow muscle contraction; little to no joint movement May require reinforcement to elicit contraction
2+	NL	Slight muscle contraction AND slight joint movement
3+	Hyperreflexia	Visible BRISK muscle contraction/moderate joint movement
4+	ABN	STRONG muscle contraction;1–3 beats of clonus
5+	ABN	STRONG muscle contraction w/sustained clonus

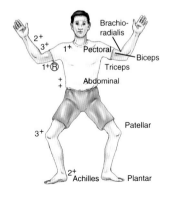

Cutaneous Reflexes

Reflex	Description	NL Response	ABN Response
Abdominal	Scratching of skin of anterior abdominal wall w/sharp object (*lateral to medial scratch* in a single dermatome). Evaluates integrity of T6–L1	Deviation of umbilicus toward stimulus	May be absent in obese patient/client or late pregnancy. Loss of reflex: corticospinal (pyramidal) system disease. Loss on one side: stroke
Cremasteric	Stroking of skin of proximal & medial aspect of thigh; involves L1, L2	Elevation of testicle in response to stroking	No response in injury to lumbosacral segments of spinal cord or lesions in pyramidal system
Bulbocavernous	Pinching of glans penis; involves S2–S4	Palpable contraction of bulbospongiosus meatus at base of penis	Lack of response w/injury to conus medullaris or sacral spinal roots
Anal sphincter	Scratching of perianal skin; involves S2–S4	Contraction of external anal sphincter	Lack of response w/injury to conus medullaris & complete SCI above L2
Plantar (most commonly tested)	Stimulus to sole of foot in sweeping motion: calcaneus → distally over shaft of 5th metatarsal → medially metatarsal heads; stimulus: even pressure for 1 sec; knee: fully extended (L5–S2)	Plantar flexion of toes produced by contraction of flexor digitorum longus, flexor hallucis longus, & lumbrical muscles of foot	Babinski response: dorsiflexion of great toe & fanning of lateral 4 toes; found in corticospinal damage

Abnormal Muscle Stretch Reflexes: Present in UMN or Frontal Lobe Damage

ABN Reflexes	Description
Jaw (cranial nerve V)	Depression of jaw slightly w/finger; percuss finger to open jaw further + reflex: jaw closes reflexively
Snout (cranial nerve VII)	Percussion of upper lip at midline in philtrum region + reflex: puckering or pursing of lips
Glabellar (cranial nerve VII)	Percussion of glabella of eye + reflex: blinking when tapped
Hoffmann (median nerves C6–C8)	Flick distal phalanx of long finger: wrist in neutral & metacarpophalangeal joint in slight extension + reflex: when thumb & index finger move toward opposition

Modified Ashworth Scale for Grading Spasticity

Grade	Description
0	No ↑ in muscle tone
1	Slight ↑ in tone; catch & release OR minimum resistance at end of ROM when moved in flexion or extension
1+	Slight ↑ in tone; catch followed by minimum resistance throughout ROM
2	Moderate ↑ in tone through most ROM, but body parts move easily
3	Considerable ↑ in tone; passive movement difficult
4	Affected part(s) rigid in flexion or extension

Tone Definitions

Abnormalities	Types	Definitions
Spasticity: velocity-dependent	Clasp: knife reflex	Passive stretch produces high resistance, followed by sudden letting go
	Clonus	Cyclical, spasmodic hyperactivity of antagonistic muscles; common in calf muscles
	Decerebrate rigidity	Sustained contraction & posturing of trunk & limbs in **full extension**; exaggerated spasticity
	Decorticate rigidity	Sustained contraction & posturing of trunk & **lower limbs** in extension & upper limbs in flexion; exaggerated form of spasticity
Rigidity: resistance uniformly ↑ in both agonist & antagonist muscles; body parts stiff and immoveable	Cogwheel rigidity	Rachet-like response to passive movement = alternate letting go & ↑ resistance to movement
	Lead pipe rigidity	Constant rigidity
Flaccidity (hypotonia): ↓ or absent muscle tone		Resistance to passive movement diminished; stretch reflexes are ↓; limbs are floppy; joints may hyperextend Weakness or paralysis: can be temporary (spinal shock) from UMN or CVA or long lasting from LMN
Dystonia: hyperkinetic movement disorder: impaired or disordered tone, sustained involuntary movements		Tone fluctuates unpredictably from low to high; dystonic posturing: sustained twisting deformity Seen in central deficit: inherited or w/neurodegenerative disorders or metabolic disorders; also seen in spasmodic torticollis (wry neck)

Tests for Autonomic Function

HR/BP	Signs of Postural Hypotension	
Bowel/bladder	Incontinence; reflexive emptying of bowel/bladder	
Signs of sympathetic hyperactivity	Excessive sweating Elevated BP Tachycardia Arrhythmias	Palpitations Flushing Nasal stuffiness Pounding headache
	Pale or mottled skin appearance; goose bumps (piloerection)	
Signs of sympathetic dystrophy (reflex sympathetic dystrophy)	Trophic changes: Change in skin & nail texture/skin color Loss of hair	Edema Lack of sweating Poor peripheral temp regulation
Observe for Horner syndrome	Miosis (papillary dilation) Ptosis (partial drooping of eyelid)	Anhydrosis (lack of sweating) Flushing of face
Observe difficulties w/swallowing	Hoarseness	
Observe for GI disturbances	Nausea, vomiting, changes in GI motility	

Upper vs. Lower Motoneuron Lesions: Signs & Symptoms

Signs & Symptoms	UMN	LMN
Paresis/plegia	Spastic	Flaccid
Deep tendon reflexes	Increased	Decreased or absent
Passive stretch response	Velocity-sensitive increase in resistance	↑ compliance of muscles
Ability to isolate muscle contractions	Loss of ability to isolate muscle contractions	Retention of ability to isolate muscle contractions
Muscle strength	Inappropriate stereotypic movement patterns w/volitional movement; muscle strength difficult to determine	Atrophy of affected muscles
Clonus	A continuous rhythmic reflex tremor initiated below an area of spinal cord injury, set in motion by reflex testing	No clonus
EMG results	Increased activity	EMG evidence of denervation
Babinski & Hoffman signs	Positive	Negative

Balance Assessment

Balance Tests and Responses

Components	Balance Responses	Tests	
Sensory elements	Detects orientation of body & body parts in reference to environment Includes: • Visual system • Somatosensory system • Vestibular system	Assess of vertigo Automatic postural reaction Crossed extensor tests Cutaneous function Flexor withdrawal Postural muscle activity Angular & linear acceleration & deceleration forces on head Righting reactions of head, trunk, limbs Visual acuity w/Snellen Eye Chart	Proprioception Regulation of muscle tone Stabilization of gaze Stretch reflex tests Visually guided movements Visual field tests
Sensory interaction	Sense of equilibrium: sense of position of center of mass in relation to support surface	Assess stand balance w/different sensory components • Surfaces: dense foam/NL/other • Visual input varies from eyes closed to open	
Musculoskeletal elements	Simple stretch reflex to functional stretch reflex to postural synergies & equilibrium reactions	ROM Tone Evaluate posture (static balance) & movement (dynamic) & response to balance disturbance	Assess for postural synergies Strength

Functional Balance Tests

Test	Description
Berg Balance Scale	Evaluates posture/control w/14 conditions: w/↓ base of support in sit/stand/single leg stance
Functional Reach Test	Evaluates ability to reach forward w/o feet moving
Timed Up and Go	Evaluates dynamic balance/mobility: timed activity of rise from chair, stand, walk 3 m, return, & sit
Balance measures: parallel, semi-tandem, tandem stand	Timed maintenance of balance during different foot positions

Functional Balance Grades

Grade	Description
NL	Able to maintain balance w/o support Accepts max challenge & shifts wt
Good	Able to maintain balance w/o support Accepts mod challenge & shifts wt but some limitations evident
Fair	Able to maintain balance w/o support Cannot tolerate challenge; cannot maintain balance w/wt shift
Poor	Requires support to maintain balance
Zero	Requires max assist to maintain balance

Berg Balance Scale	
Components	**Scoring**
1. Sitting to standing Please stand up. Try not to use your hands for support.	Able to stand, not using hands = 4 Able to stand using hands = 3 Able to stand w/hands & several tries = 2 Needs min assist to stand and stabilize = 1 Needs mod or max assist to stand = 0
2. Standing unsupported Stand for 2 min w/o holding on to support.	Able to stand safely for 2 min = 4 Able to stand for 2 min w/supervision = 3 Able to stand for 30 sec, unsupported = 2 Needs several tries to stand for 30 sec, unsupported = 1 Unable to stand for 30 sec, unassisted = 0
3. Sitting unsupported, w/feet on floor Sit w/arms folded for 2 min.	Able to sit safely & securely for 2 min = 4 Able to sit for 2 min under supervision = 3 Able to sit for 30 sec = 2 Able to sit for 10 sec = 1 Unable to sit unsupported = 0
4. Standing to sitting Please sit down.	Sits safely w/minimal use of hands = 4 Controls descent by using hands = 3 Uses backs of legs against chair to control descent = 2 Sits independently but has uncontrolled descent = 1 Needs assist to sit down = 0
5. Transfers Please move from chair to bed and back again. One way toward a seat w/armrests One way toward a seat w/o armrest	Able to transfer w/min use of hands = 4 Able to transfer w/full use of hands = 3 Able to transfer w/cueing &/or sup = 2 Needs assist of one person = 1 Needs assist of 2 to transfer safely/unable to transfer = 0

Continued

Berg Balance Scale—cont'd

Components	Scoring
6. Standing unsupported w/eyes closed Close your eyes and stand still for 10 seconds.	Able to stand still for 10 sec = 4 Able to stand still for 10 sec w/sup = 3 Able to stand still for 3 sec = 2 Unable to keep eyes closed for 3 sec = 1 Needs help to keep from falling = 0
7. Standing unsupported w/feet together Place your feet together and stand without holding on to support.	Able to place feet together & stand 1 min = 4 Able to place feet together & stand for 1 min w/supervision = 3 Able to place feet together/unable to hold for 30 sec = 2 Needs help to attain position, but able to stand for 15 sec = 1 Needs help to attain position, & unable to hold for 15 sec = 0
8. Reaching forward w/outstretched arm Lift arms to 90°. Examiner places ruler at the fingertips when arm is at 90°. Stretch out your fingers and reach forward as far as you can. Do not move your feet. When possible use both arms to avoid rotation of trunk.	Can reach forward confidently more than 10 in = 4 Can reach forward more than 5 in = 3 Can reach forward more than 2 inches = 2 Reaches forward, but needs supervision = 1 Needs help to keep from falling = 0

Berg Balance Scale—cont'd

Components	Scoring
9. Picking up item from floor Pick up the shoe/slipper, which is placed in front of you on the floor.	Able to pick up the slipper safely & easily = 4 Able to pick up the slipper, but needs supervision, & keeps balance independently = 3 Unable to pick up the slipper, reaches 2–3 in from it = 2 Unable to pick up the slipper, & needs supervision when trying = 1 Unable to pick up the slipper, & needs assist to keep from falling = 0
10. Turning to look behind over left and right shoulder Turn to look behind you over your left shoulder, and then repeat over your right shoulder.	Looks behind from both sides & shifts weight well = 4 Looks behind to one side only, other side shows less weight shift = 3 Turns sideways only, but maintains balance = 2 Needs supervision when turning = 1 point Needs assist to keep from falling = 0
11. Turning through 360° Turn around completely in a full circle one way, pause, and then turn a full circle in the opposite direction.	Able to turn through 360° safely each way in <4 sec = 4 Able to turn through 360° safely to one side in <4 sec = 3 Able to turn through 360° safely but slowly = 2 Needs close supervision or verbal cueing = 1 Needs assist while turning = 0
12. Number of times stool touched while stepping Place each foot alternately on the stool. Continue until each foot has touched the stool four times.	Able to stand independently & safely & complete 8 steps in 20 sec = 4 Able to stand independently & complete 8 steps in 20 sec = 3 Able to complete 4 steps, w/o aid, w/ supervision = 2 Able to complete >2 steps, needs min assist = 1 Needs assist to keep from falling/unable to try = 0

Continued

Components	Scoring
13. Standing unsupported w/one foot in front of the other (Demonstrate this to subject first.) Place one foot in front of the other. If you feel that you cannot place your foot directly in front, try to step far enough ahead for the heel of your forward foot to be in front of the toes of the other foot.	Able to place feet in tandem independently & hold for 30 sec = 4 Able to place one foot in front of the other independently & hold for 30 sec = 3 Able to take small step independently & hold for 30 sec = 2 Needs help to step, but can hold for 15 sec = 1 Loses balance while stepping or standing = 0
14. Standing on one leg Stand on one leg for as long as you can w/o holding on.	Able to lift leg independently & hold for 10 sec = 4 Able to lift leg independently & hold for 5–10 sec = 3 Able to lift leg for more than 3 sec = 2 Tries to lift leg, unable to hold for 3 sec, but remains standing independently = 1 Unable to try, or needs assist to prevent falling = 0

Berg Balance Scale Score	Falls Risk	
41–56	LOW	
21–40	MEDIUM	
0–20	HIGH	Total score (maximum possible score = 56)

Reproduced with the permission of Dr KO Berg from Berg KO, Wood-Dauphinee SL, Williams JI et al. Measuring balance in the elderly: preliminary development of an instrument. Physiother Can. 1989; 41: 304–11.

Tinetti Balance and Gait Tests

Balance Assessment

Activity	Description	Score
1. Sitting balance	Leans or slides in chair	0
	Steady and safe	1
2. Arises	Unable to arise w/o help	0
	Able to arise, uses arms to help	2
	Able to arise w/o arms	2
3. Attempts to arise	Unable to attempt to arise w/o help	0
	Able to arise, requires >1 attempt	1
	Able to arise in 1 attempt	2
4. Immediate standing balance (first 5 sec)	Unsteady (swaggers, moves feet, sways)	0
	Steady, but uses support or walker	1
	Steady w/o walker or support	2
5. Standing balance	Unsteady	0
	Steady, wide stance (>4 in heels apart) & uses cane or other support	1
	Narrow stance w/o support	2
6. Nudged while feet close together: light push	Begins to fall	0
	Staggers, grabs, catches self	1
	Steady	2
7. Eyes closed, feet close	Unsteady	0
	Steady	1
8. Turning through 360°	Discontinuous steps	0
	Continuous steps	1
	Unsteady (grabs or staggers)	0
	Steady	1
9. Sitting down	Unsafe (falls, misjudges distance)	0
	Uses arms or not smooth motion	1
	Safe, smooth motion	2
Balance Score	**Out of 16**	

Continued

Gait Assessment

10. Initiation of gait after subject told "GO"	Any hesitancy or multiple attempts	0
	No hesitancy	1
11. Step length and height	R swing foot does not pass L stance foot	0
	R foot passes L stance foot	1
	R foot does not clear the floor completely	0
	R foot completely clears floor	1
	L swing foot does not pass R stance	0
	L foot passes R foot stance	1
	Left foot does not clear floor	0
	Left foot completely clears floor	1
12. Step symmetry	R & L step length not equal	0
	R & L step length appear equal	1
13. Step continuity	Stopping or discontinuous bet steps	0
	Steps appear continuous	1
14. Path: observe excursion of 1 foot over 10 foot course	Marked deviation	0
	Mild/mod deviation or uses walk aid	1
	Straight w/o walk aid	2
15. Trunk	Marked sway or uses walking aid	0
	No sway, knees flexed or hyperextended, or arms spread	1
	No sway, no flexion, no arms spread	2
16. Walking Stance	Heels apart	0
	Heels almost touching while walking	1
	Gait Score: Out of 12	
	Total Balance and Gait: Out of 28	

Tinetti Total Score	≤18	19–23	≥24
Risk of Falls	High	Moderate	Low

Reproduced with the permission of Mary Tinetti from Tinetti ME. Performance-oriented assessment of mobility problems in elderly patients. *J Am Geriatr Soc.* 1986; 34: 119–26.

Romberg Balance Test

Patient/client stands w/feet parallel and together (some say w/arms folded across chest). Close eyes for 20–30 sec. Judge the amount of sway or time position held.

Abnormal test: Eyes open, loss of balance, stepping during test.

Clinical Test of Sensory Interaction and Balance

Observe patient/client's attempt to maintain balance while standing w/feet together hands on hips or w/hands across waist for 30 sec under conditions 1–6 below. SHOES REMOVED

Condition	Time
1. Eyes open, firm surface	___/30 sec
2. Eyes closed, firm surface	___/30 sec
3. Eyes open w/visual conflict dome, firm surface	___/30 sec
4. Eyes open, compliant surface	___/30 sec
5. Eyes closed, compliant surface	___/30 sec
6. Eyes open w/visual conflict dome, compliant surface	___/30 sec

Modified Clinical Test of Sensory Interaction on Balance (mCTSIB)

Patient/client stands w/feet together and hands on hips or across abdomen for 30 sec. Proceed to next condition when one 30-sec trial is completed or all three trials are performed. SHOES REMOVED

Condition	Time
Eyes open, firm surface	1st: ___/30 sec 2nd: ___/30 sec 3rd: ___/30 sec Mean score _____
Eyes closed, firm surface	1st: ___/30 sec 2nd: ___/30 sec 3rd: ___/30 sec Mean score _____
Eyes open, foam surface	1st: ___/30 sec 2nd: ___/30 sec 3rd: ___/30 sec Mean score _____

Continued

Modified Clinical Test of Sensory Interaction on Balance (mCTSIB)—cont'd

Condition	Time
Eyes closed, foam surface	1st: ___/30 sec 2nd: ___/30 sec 3rd: ___/30 sec Mean score _____

TOTAL SCORE: ___/120 sec (mean score used for each condition if >1 trial is performed)

Full Stance/Semi-Tandem/Tandem Balance Test

Patient/client should remain in position for 10 sec before moving on to next position. Shoes off. No support allowed. When patient/client moves out of position, record time.

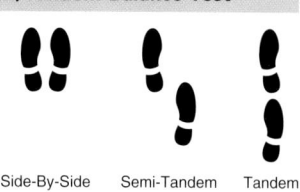

Side-By-Side   Semi-Tandem   Tandem

Timed Single Leg Stance

Procedure

Shoes off, stand on one leg, place arms across chest w/hands touching shoulders. Look straight ahead w/eyes open & focus on object 3 ft ahead. Should maintain 10 sec.

Shoes off, stand on one leg w/eyes closed for 10 sec.

Older adults: 89% of time can maintain for 10 sec.
Nursing home patient/clients: 45% of time can maintain for 10 sec.
From Bohannon R. *Phys Ther* 1984 64(7):1067

Functional Reach Test: Voluntary Postural Control

Procedure

Attach a yardstick to wall at level of patient/client's acromion process. Patient/client stands w/feet shoulder width apart and arm raised to 90° (parallel to floor, palm facing medially). Instruct patient/client to reach as far forward as possible w/o letting feet rise off floor or hand touch yardstick. Location of middle finger is recorded.

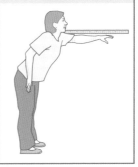

Healthy individuals w/adequate functional balance can reach 10 in. Scores ≤6 indicate limited functional balance.

Duncan, P. W., D. K. Weiner, et al. (1990). "Functional reach: a new clinical measure of balance." *J Gerontol* **45**(6): M192–197

Multidirectional Reach Test

Patient/client reaches forward, to the right, to the left, & leans backward. The distance reached is measured. Normative values as follows:

Forward reach	8.9 in	Reach to left	6.6 in
Backward reach	4.6 in	Reach to right	6.8 in

Performance-Oriented Mobility Assessment (POMA)

Activity	Scoring
1. Sitting down in armless chair against a wall	0 = unable w/o help or collapses (plops) on or lands off center of chair 1 = able & does not meet criteria of 0 or 2 2 = sits in smooth, safe motion centered
2. Sitting balance	0 = unable to maintain position 1 = leans slightly or slight distance from back of chair 2 = steady, safe, upright
3. Arising	0 = unable w/o help or loses balance or requires >3 attempts 1 = able but requires 3 attempts 2 = able in ≤2 attempts
4. Immediate standing balance (first 5 sec)	0 = unsteady, staggering, moves feet, trunk sway, grabs objects 1 = steady but uses walker or cane or mild staggering, no grabbing objects 2 = steady w/o walker or cane or support
5. Stand	0 = unable or unsteady or holds ≤3 sec 1 = able but uses cane, walker, or other support for 4–9 sec 2 = narrow stance w/o support for 10 sec
6. Pull test: examiner stands behind and exerts mild pull back at waist	0 = begins to fall 1 = takes more than 2 steps back 2 = fewer than 2 steps backward and steady
7. Able to stand on right leg unsupported	0 = unable or holds <3 sec or holds on to objects 1 = able to stand 3–4 sec 2 = able to stand 5 sec

Performance-Oriented Mobility Assessment (POMA)—cont'd

Activity	Scoring
8. Walks down 10-ft walkway, turns, and walks back (use walk aid if usually uses walk aid)	Type of surface 1 = linoleum or tile 2 = wood 3 = cement 4 = other
9. Initiation of gait (after told "GO")	0 = any hesitancy or multiple attempts to start 1 = no hesitancy
10. Side-by-side standing balance	1 = mild or mod deviation or uses walk aid 2 = straight w/o walk aid
11. Missed step (trip or loss of balance)	0 = yes, and would have fallen, or more than 2 missed steps 1 = yes, but appropriate attempt to recover and no more than 2 missed steps 2 = none
12. Turning while walking	0 = almost falls 1 = mild staggering but catches self, uses walker or cane 2 = steady, w/o walk aid
13. Step over obstacles (place 2 shoes on course 4 ft apart)	0 = begins to fall or unable or walks around obstacle, or >2 missed steps 1 = able to step over obstacles but some staggering and catches self or 1–2 missed steps 2 = able & steady at stepping over all 4 obstacles w/no missed steps

Reproduced with the permission of Mary Tinetti from Tinetti, Mary E. Performance-oriented assessment of mobility problems in elderly patients. *J Am Geriatr Soc.*, Vol 34(2), Feb 1986, 119–126.

Coordination Tests

Test	Description	Abnormalities
Alternate heel to knee or toe	Supine: touch knee & big toe alternately w/heel of opposite extremity	Cerebellar dysfunction: slow/dysrhythmic
Alternate nose to finger	Sitting: touch tip of nose & tip of therapist's finger w/index finger; change position of therapist's finger	Cerebellar dysfunction: ataxic, slow
Draw a circle	Patient/client draws imaginary circle in air w/upper or lower extremity; may be performed supine	Cerebellar disease: ataxic, slow
Finger to finger	Shoulders abducted to 90° w/elbows extended; patient/client brings both index fingers to midline & touches fingers	Slow w/intention tremors
Finger to nose	Shoulders abducted to 90° w/elbows extended; patient/client brings tip of index finger to tip of nose	Cerebellar disease: unsteady or shaky movements; action or intention tremors
Finger opposition	Tip of thumb pressed to tip of each finger in sequence; ↑ speed gradually	Dysdiadochokinesia: inability to perform rapid contraction/relaxation
Finger to therapist's finger	Sitting opposite, therapist holds finger in front of patient/client, who is required to touch finger as therapist moves finger around	Slow or dysrhythmic
Rebound test	Elbow flex: therapist applies manual resistance to produce isometric contraction of biceps: resistance suddenly released	Opposing muscle group (triceps) does not contract and "check" movement

Coordination Tests—cont'd

Test	Description	Abnormalities
Pronation/ supination	Elbows flexed to 90° & held close to body Patient/client alternately turns palms up & down ↑ speed gradually	Slow or dysrhythmic
Tapping foot	Taps ball of foot on floor w/o raising knee; heel keeps contact w/floor	Slow movement, unable to hold heel on floor
Tapping hand	W/elbow flexed, forearm pronated, patient/client taps hand on knee	Slow movement, unable to perform rapid tapping
Fixation or hold position	UE: patient/client holds arms horizontally in front LE: patient/client holds knee in extended position	Unable to hold arms or knees in position; ataxic movements

Dynamic Gait Index

Mark lowest category

Category	Instructions	Scoring
Gait level surface	Walk at normal speed from start to 20 ft	3 = walks 20 ft w/o assist device 2 = mild impairment. Walks 20 ft, uses assistive devices, slower speed, mild gait deviations. 1 = mod impairment; walks 20 ft slow speed, abnormal gait pattern, evidence for imbalance. 0 = severe impairment; cannot walk 20 ft w/o assist, severe gait deviations, or imbalance

Continued

Mark lowest category

Category	Instructions	Scoring
Change in gait speed	Begin walking at normal pace for 5 ft, when instructed, walk fast for 5 ft, when instructed, walk slowly for 5 ft	3 = **Normal:** Able to smoothly change walking speed w/o loss of balance or gait deviation. Shows difference between gait speeds 2 = **Mild impairment:** Able to change speed but mild gait deviations, or unable to achieve a change in velocity, or uses an assistive device 1 = **Mod impairment:** Minimal changes in walk speed, or shows gait deviations, or loses balance but is able to recover & continue walking 0 = **Severe impairment:** Cannot change speeds, or loses balance & has to reach for wall or be caught
Gait w/ horizontal head turns	Begin walking at your normal pace. When I tell you to "look right," keep walking straight, but turn your head to the right. Keep looking to the right until I tell you to "look left," then keep walking straight and turn your head to the left. Keep your head to the left until I tell you to "look straight," then keep walking straight but return your head to the center.	3 = **Normal** 2 = **Mild impairment:** Performs head turns smoothly w/slight change in gait velocity or uses walking aid 1 = **Mod impairment:** Performs head turns w/moderate change in gait velocity, slows down, staggers but recovers; can continue to walk 0 = **Severe impairment:** Performs task w/severe disruptions of gait (ie, staggers outside path, loses balance, stops, reaches for wall)

Dynamic Gait Index—cont'd

Mark lowest category

Category	Instructions	Scoring
Gait w/ vertical head turns	Begin walking at your normal pace. When I tell you to "look up," keep walking straight, but tip your head and look up. Keep looking up until I tell you to "look down," then keep walking straight and turn your head down. Keep looking down until I tell you to "look straight," then keep walking straight but return your head to the center.	3 = **Normal:** Performs head turns w/no change in gait 2 = **Mild impairment:** Performs task w/ slight change in gait velocity (ie, minor disruption to smooth gait path or uses walking aid) 1 = **Mod impairment:** Performs tasks w/moderate change in gait velocity, slows down, staggers but recovers; can continue to walk 0 = **Severe impairment:** Performs task w/severe disruption or gait (ie, staggers outside path, loses balance, stops, reaches for wall)
Gait and pivot turn	Begin walking at your normal pace. When I tell you to "stop and turn," turn as quickly as you can to face the opposite direction and stop.	3 = **Normal:** Pivots & turns safely within 3 sec & stops quickly 2 = **Mild impairment:** Pivots & turns safely in >3 sec & stops; no loss of balance 1 = **Mod impairment:** Turns slowly, requires verbal cueing, requires several small steps to catch balance following turn & stop 0 = **Severe impairment:** Cannot turn safely, requires assist to turn & stop

Continued

Dynamic Gait Index—cont'd

Mark lowest category

Category	Instructions	Scoring
Step over obstacle	Begin walking at your normal speed. When you come to the shoebox, step over it, not around it, and keep walking.	3 = **Normal:** Able to step over box w/o changing gait speed; no imbalance 2 = **Mild impairment:** Able to step over box, but must slow down & adjust steps 1 = **Mod impairment:** Able to step over box but must stop, then step over. May require verbal cueing 0 = **Severe impairment:** Cannot perform w/o assist
Step around obstacles	Begin walking at your normal speed. When you come to the first cone (6 ft away), walk around the right side of it. When you come to the second cone (6 ft past first cone), walk around it to the left.	3 = **Normal:** Able to walk around cones safely w/o changing speed; good balance 2 = **Mild impairment:** Able to step around both cones, but must slow down & adjust steps to clear cones 1 = **Mod impairment:** Able to clear cones, but must slow speed to accomplish task, or requires verbal cueing 0 = **Severe impairment:** Unable to clear cones, walks into one or both cones, or requires physical assist
Stairs	Walk up these stairs as you would at home (ie, using the rail if necessary). At the top, turn around and walk down.	3 = **Normal:** Alternating feet, no rail. 2 = **Mild impairment:** Alternating feet, must use rail. 1 = **Mod impairment:** 2 feet to stair, must use rail 0 = **Severe impairment:** Cannot do safely

(Adapted from Shumway-Cook A, Wollacott M. Motor Control: Theory and Practical Applications. Baltimore: Williams and Wilkins, 1995).

Neurodiagnostics

Diagnostic Tests/ Indications	Information From Tests	Precautions/Notes
Clinical EMG Needle insertion for single motor unit potentials; to study motor unit activity & integrity of neuromuscular system; identifies denervated areas of muscle and myopathic changes	Records electrical activity present in contracting muscle Identifies LMN disorders & nerve root compression & distinguishes neurogenic from myopathic disorders	Examiner judges patient/ client effort: determines if recruit is NL Inaccurate placement: distorts recorded potentials Interpretation problems w/anatomical anomalies: accuracy improves w/experience in interpretation
Kinesiological EMG To examine muscle function during specific purposeful tasks	Patterns of muscle response, onset & cessation of activity & level of response Used to facilitate or inhibit specific muscle activity	Compare information gathered from nerve conduction velocity Same precautions as clinical EMG
Nerve conduction velocity Uses surface electrodes; to assess peripheral nerves: sensory and motor	Evaluation of peripheral neuropathies, motoneuron disease, demyelinating disorders	Routine testing does not pick up peripheral nerve disorder affecting small unmyelinated C fibers **Early** peripheral neuropathy may show absent sensory but NL motor
EEG To assess any brain dysfunction, especially epilepsy	Differential Dx of seizures: especially if spontaneous attack; no EEG activity: Dx of brain death	Sensitive but not specific; inexpensive
Magnetoencephalography (MEG) to assess any brain dysfunction: epilepsy	NEW: records magnetic field produced by brain's electrical activity	Better than EEG: brain mapping; localizes regions affected by pathology prior to surgical removal

Continued

Neurodiagnostics—cont'd

Diagnostic Tests/Indications	Information From Tests	Precautions/Notes
CT scan To identify structural diseases of brain & spinal cord	Diagnostic test of choice for evaluation of disease of brain/spine associated w/acute trauma, intra- or subarachnoid hemorrhage, bony lesions of skull, cervical/lumbar root lesions, & brachial or lumbosacral plexus lesions	Expensive; cannot diagnose metabolic or inflammatory disorders. Used instead of MRI in presence of metal, including pacemaker or cerebral aneurysm clips; or if patient/client agitated or claustrophobic
Magnetic resonance imaging	A magnetic field & pulses of radio wave energy take pictures of the head. The MRI can show tissue damage or disease, such as infection, inflammation, or a tumor. In the brain T_1-weighted scans provide good gray matter/white matter contrast; in other words, T_1-weighted images highlight fat deposition.	Precautions w/metal, implants, pacemakers, & if patient/client is claustrophobic
Lumbar puncture To confirm suspicion of CNS infection; before anticoagulant therapy for cerebrovascular disease	Cell count & differential Cytological exam for neoplastic cells Stains for bacteria & fungi Culture for organisms	Contraindicated if tissue infection in region of puncture site Complications of test: headache & backache
Angiography To visualize blood vessels of brain & spinal cord	Evaluate cerebrovascular disease, cerebral venous sinuses, intracranial aneurysms, & spinal A-V anomalies	Evaluate patient/client for contrast dye allergies

Neuromuscular Interventions

Procedural Interventions	Specific Activities	
Balance, coordination, & agility training	Developmental activities training Motor control & learning training/retraining Neuromuscular education/re-education Perceptual training	Postural awareness training Sensory training/retraining Task-specific performance training Vestibular training
Body mechanics & postural stabilization	Body mechanics training Postural control training	Postural stabilization activities Posture awareness training
Gait and locomotion training	Developmental activities training Gait training	Perceptual training Wheelchair training
Neuromotor development training	Motor training Movement pattern training	
Flexibility exercises	Muscle lengthening & stretching; ROM exercises	
Strength, power, & endurance training	Active assistive, active resistive exercises (concentric/eccentric, isokinetic, isometric, isotonic) Task-specific performance training	
Electrotherapeutic modalities	Biofeedback Electrical stimulation	
Physical agents & mechanical modalities	Pulsed electromagnetic fields Cryotherapy Hydrotherapy Light: infrared/laser/ultraviolet Sound: phonophoresis/ultrasound Thermotherapy: diathermy/dry heat/hot packs/paraffin Compression therapies: bandaging/garments/taping/contact casting/vasopneumatic compression Gravity-assisted compression devices: stand/tilt table CPM traction devices: intermittent/positional/sustained	

Continued

Neuromuscular Interventions—cont'd

Procedural Interventions	Specific Activities
Functional training in self-care & home management	ADL training Barrier accommodations/modifications Device/equipment use & training Functional training programs: back school, simulated environments, task adaptation, travel training IADL training Injury prevention or reduction
Functional training in work, community, & leisure	Same as self-care & home management but in work, community, or leisure setting

Special Considerations/Populations

Spinal Cord Injury

American Spinal Injury Association Classification

Impairment Scale	Description
A: Complete transaction of spinal cord	No motor or sensory function is preserved in the sacral segments S4–S5
B: Incomplete	Sensory but not motor is preserved below neurological level
C: Incomplete	Motor function preserved below neurological level: > half of key muscles below neurological level have < grade 3
D: Incomplete	Motor function preserved below neurological level, at least half of key muscles below neurological level have a muscle grade = or >3
E: NL	Motor and sensory function are NL

Potential Problems w/Spinal Cord Injury

Problem	Symptoms	Description
Autonomic dysreflexia	Hypertension Bradycardia Profuse sweating ↑ spasticity Headache Vasodilation above lesion Goose bumps	Pathological reflex in lesions above T6; episodes ↓ over time; rare after 3 y post injury Acute onset from noxious stimuli below level of injury: bladder distention, rectal distention, pressure sores, urinary stones, bladder infection, noxious cutaneous stimuli, kidney malfunction, environmental temperature changes Treatment: medical emergency: assess catheter for kinks; change position; assess source of irritation: bladder irrigation or bowel
Postural hypotension	↓ in BP w/ change in position to upright	Loss of sympathetic vasoconstriction control associated w/lack of muscle tone, > in cervical & upper thoracic lesions Develop edema in legs, ankles, & feet. Treatment: adapt to vertical position slowly, compress stockings & abdominal binder, meds to ↑ BP, diuretics to ↓ edema
Heterotopic bone formation	Loss of ROM	Osteogenesis (bone formation) in soft tissues below level of lesion: extra-capsular and extra-articular Problems w/joint motion & function Treatment: drugs; physical therapy for ROM; surgery
Contractures	Severe limitations in ROM	Develops secondary to position: prolonged shortening Causes: lack of active muscle, gravity, positioning
DVT	Local swelling, erythema, & heat	Thrombus (clot) develops in vein; may travel to lungs: ↑ risk of pulmonary embolus & cardiac arrest Treatment: anticoagulation (heparin first)

Continued

Potential Problems w/Spinal Cord Injury—cont'd

Problem	Symptoms	Description
Osteoporosis renal calculi	Stone formation Fracture, postural changes	Net loss of bone mass; ↑ risk for fracture: ↑ estimated risk first 6 mo; post injury ↑ Ca++ in blood; ↑ risk of stone formation
Pressure sores	Erythema, skin breakdown	Ulcerations of soft tissue: from pressure (wt)

Spinal Cord Injury Bowel & Bladder Changes

Dysfunction	Bowel	Bladder	Sexual Functioning
Spinal shock	No reflexive movement	Flaccid: no tone	No reflexes seen
UMN	Reflex bowel: responds to digital stimulation	Contract/reflex empty in response to level of filling pressure Reflex arc intact Intermittent catheterization usually used	**M:** Reflexogenic erectile function (only 3% ejaculate) **F:** Reflexogenic sexual arousal (lubrication, engorgement, clitoral erection) Fertility/pregnancy unimpaired, often early labor
LMN	Autonomous/nonreflex bowel: relies on straining & manual evacuation	Nonreflex bladder: flaccid Emptied by ↑ intra-abdominal pressure/Crede maneuver & timed voiding	**M:** Often no erections 25% psychogenic erections 15% ejaculate **F:** No reflex sexual arousal: + psychogenic responses Fertility/pregnancy unimpaired, often early labor
Incomplete	Usually similar to complete UMN	Usually similar to complete UMN	**M:** 98% reflexogenic erectile function **F:** Reflexogenic sexual arousal

Communication Disorders

Disorder	Description
Aphasia Anomic	Difficulty naming objects; word-finding problems
Broca	Difficulty expressing, mild difficulty understanding complex syntax
Conduction	Difficulty in repetition of spoken language; word-finding pauses & letter or whole word substitutions
Crossed	Transient; occurs in RH persons w/R hemisphere lesion; ↓ comprehension
Global	Most common & severe form; spontaneous speech: few stereotypical words/sounds; comprehension ↓ or absent; repetition, reading, & writing: impaired
Subcortical (thalamic)	Dysarthria & mild anomia w/comprehension deficits; in lesions of thalamus, putamen, caudate, or int cap
Transcortical	Spontaneous speech restricted: able to repeat, comprehend, & read well
Wernecke	Severe disturbance in auditory comprehension w/inappropriate responses to questions
Agraphia	Writing ability disturbed; associated w/aphasia; found in lesions in post-language area or frontal language area
Aprosody	Disturbance of melodic qualities of language; change in intonation patterns or expressive language
Dysarthria	Result from loss of control of muscles of articulation

Sydney Swallowing Questionnaire

Question	No Difficulty to Swallow	In Between	Unable to Swallow at All
1. How much **difficulty** do you have swallowing at present?			
2. How much difficulty do you have swallowing **THIN liquids**? (eg, tea, soft drinks, beer, coffee)			
3. How much difficulty do you have swallowing **THICK liquids**? (eg, milkshakes, soups, custard)			
4. How much difficulty do you have swallowing **SOFT foods**? (eg, Mornays, scrambled egg, mashed potato)			
5. How much difficulty do you have swallowing **HARD foods**? (eg, steak, raw fruit, raw vegetables)			
6. How much difficulty do you have swallowing **DRY foods**? (eg, bread, biscuits, nuts)			
7. Do you have any difficulty **swallowing your saliva**?			
8. Do you have any difficulty **starting a swallow**?			

Sydney Swallowing Questionnaire—cont'd

	Never Occurs	In Between	Occurs Every Time
9. Do you ever have a **feeling of food** getting **stuck** in your throat when you swallow?			
10. Do you ever **cough or choke** when swallowing **solid foods**? (eg, bread, meat or fruit)			
11. Do you ever **cough or choke** when swallowing **liquids**? (eg, coffee, tea, water, beer)			
12. How long does it take you to **eat an average meal**? Please **TICK ONE**. Less than **15** min ____ About **15–30** min ____ About **30–45** min ____ About **45–60** min ____ More than **60** min ____ **Unable** to swallow at all _			
13. When you swallow, does food or liquid **go up behind your nose or come out of your nose**?			
14. Do you ever need to **swallow more than once** for your food to go down?			
15. Do you ever **cough up or spit out food or liquids DURING a meal**?			
16. How do you rate the **severity** of your swallowing problem today?	No problem		Extreme problem
17. How **much** does your swallowing problem **interfere w/your enjoyment or quality of life**?	No interference		Extreme interference

Drooling Severity and Frequency Scale

Drooling Severity Scale	Never drools, dry	1
	Mild: drooling, only lips wet	2
	Moderate: drool reaches the lips & chin	3
	Severe: drool drips off chin & on to clothing	4
	Profuse: drooling off the body & on to objects (furniture, books)	5
Drooling Frequency Scale	1 = No drooling	1
	2 = Occasionally drools	2
	3 = Frequently drools	4
	4 = Constant drooling	4

The Drooling Score equals the sum of the Severity and Frequency sub-scores.

Flexion and Extension Synergy

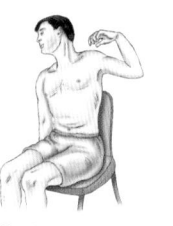

Flexion synergy.

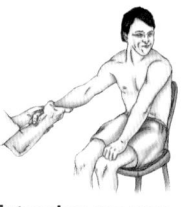

Extension synergy.

Indicators for Poor Recovery Post Stroke

1. Decreased alertness, inattention, poor memory, & inability to learn new tasks or follow simple commands _____
2. Severe neglect or agnosia _____
3. Significant medical problems, especially CV or DJD _____

4. Serious language disturbances _____
5. Less well defined social & economic problems _____

Synergy Patterns in Stroke

	Flexion Synergy Components	Extension Synergy Components
Upper extremity	Scapular retraction/elevation or hyperextension	Scapular protraction
	Shoulder abduction/external rotation	Shoulder adduction*/internal rotation
	Elbow flexion*	Elbow extension
	Forearm supination	Forearm pronation*
	Wrist & finger flexion	Wrist & finger flexion
Lower extremity	Hip flexion,* abduction, external rotation	Hip extension, adduction*, internal rotation
	Knee flexion	Knee extension*
	Ankle dorsiflexion, inversion	Ankle plantar flexion*, inversion
	Toe dorsiflexion	Toe plantar flexion

*Strongest component.

Guide to PT Practice Patterns for Neurological Impairments

Preferred Practice	Includes
Pattern 5A: Primary prevention/risk reduction for loss of balance and falling	Advanced age, alteration to senses, dementia, depression, dizziness, Hx of falls, meds, musculoskeletal diseases, neuromuscular diseases, prolonged inactivity, vestibular pathology
Pattern 5B: Impaired neuromotor development	Alteration in senses, birth trauma, cognitive delay, genetic syndromes, developmental coordination disorder, developmental delay, dyspraxia, fetal alcohol syndrome, prematurity

Continued

Preferred Practice	Includes
Pattern 5C: Impaired motor function & sensory integrity associated w/nonprogressive CNS disorders: congenital origin or acquired in infancy or childhood	Brain anoxia/hypoxia, birth trauma, brain anomalies, cerebral palsy, encephalitis, premature birth, traumatic brain injury, genetic syndromes (w/CNS), hydrocephalus, infectious disease (w/CNS), meningocele, neoplasm, tethered cord
Pattern 5D: Impaired motor function & sensory integrity associated w/nonprogressive CNS disorders acquired in adolescence or adulthood	Aneurysm, brain anoxia/hypoxia, Bell palsy, CVA, infectious disease (affects CNS), intracranial neurosurgical procedure, neoplasm, seizures, traumatic brain injury
Pattern 5E: Impaired motor function & sensory integrity associated w/progressive CNS disorders	AIDS, alcoholic ataxia, Alzheimer diseases, ALS, basal ganglia disease, cerebellar ataxia, cerebellar disease, idiopathic progressive cortical disease, intracranial neurosurgical procedures, Huntington disease, multiple sclerosis, neoplasm, Parkinson disease, primary lateral palsy, progressive muscular atrophy, seizures
Pattern 5F Impaired peripheral nerve integrity & muscle performance associated w/peripheral nerve injury	Neuropathies: carpal or cubital tunnel syndrome, Erb palsy, radial or tarsal tunnel syndrome; peripheral vestibular disorders: labyrinthitis, paroxysmal positional vertigo; surgical nerve lesions, traumatic nerve lesions
Pattern 5G: Impaired motor function & sensory integrity associated w/acute or chronic polyneuropathies	Amputation, Guillain-Barré syndrome, postpolio syndrome, axonal polyneuropathies: alcoholic, diabetic, renal, ANS dysfunction, leprosy

Preferred Practice	Includes
Pattern 5H: Impaired motor function, peripheral nerve integrity, & sensory integrity associated w/nonprogressive disorders of the spinal cord	Benign spinal neoplasm, complete/incomplete spinal cord lesions, Infectious diseases of spinal cord, spinal cord compression: degenerative spinal joint disease, herniated disk, osteomyelitis, spondylosis.
Pattern 5I: Impaired arousal, ROM, & motor control associated w/ coma, near coma, or vegetative state	Brain anoxia, birth trauma, CVA, infectious/inflammatory disease affecting CNS, neoplasm, premature birth, traumatic brain injury

From APTA: Guide to Physical Therapist Practice, 2nd ed. Physical Therapy, 2003;81:9–744.

M00–M99 Diseases of the Musculoskeletal System and Connective Tissue

M00–M25 Arthropathies

M00–M03	Infectious arthropathies
M05–M14	Inflammatory polyarthropathies
M15–M19	Arthrosis
M20–M25	Other joint disorders

M30–M36 Systemic Connective Tissue Disorders

M40–M54 Dorsopathies

M40–M43	Deforming dorsopathies
M45–M49	Spondylopathies
M50–M54	Other dorsopathies

M60–M79 Soft Tissue Disorders

M60–M63	Disorders of muscles
M65–M68	Disorders of synovium and tendon
M70–M79	Other soft tissue disorders

M80–M94 Osteopathies and Chondropathies

M80–M85	Disorders of bone density and structure
M86–M90	Other osteopathies
M91–M94	Chondropathies

M95–M99 Other Disorders of the Musculoskeletal System and Connective Tissue

R25–R29 Symptoms and Signs Involving the Nervous and Musculoskeletal Systems

R25	Abnormal involuntary movements
R26	Abnormalities of gait and mobility
R27	Other and unspecified lack of coordination
R29	Other symptoms and signs involving the nervous and musculoskeletal systems

S00–T07 Injuries

S10–S19	Injuries to the neck
S20–S29	Injuries to the thorax
S30–S39	Injuries to the abdomen, lower back, lumbar spine, and pelvis
S40–S49	Injuries to the shoulder and upper arm
S50–S59	Injuries to the elbow and forearm
S60–S69	Injuries to the wrist and hand
S70–S79	Injuries to the hip and thigh

S80–S89 Injuries to the knee and lower leg
S90–S99 Injuries to the ankle and foot
T00–T07 Injuries involving multiple body regions
T08–T14 Injuries to unspecified part of trunk, limb, or body region

V01–X59 Accidents

From World Health Organization. International Statistical Classification of Diseases, ed. 10. http://apps.who.int/classifications/icd10/browse/2010/en with permission.

Musculoskeletal Assessment

Musculoskeletal Quick Screen

Upper Quarter Screening Exam	Normal	ABN
1. Posture assessment		
2. Active ROM cervical spine		
3. Passive overpressures if symptom free		
4. Resisted muscle tests cervical spine (rotation C1)		
5. Resisted shoulder elevation (C2, C3, C4)		
6. Resisted shoulder abduction (C5)		
7. Active shoulder flexion & rotations		
8. Resisted elbow flexion (C6)		
9. Resisted elbow extension (C7)		
10. Active ROM elbow		
11. Resisted wrist flexion (C7)		
12. Resisted wrist extension (C6)		
13. Resisted thumb extension (C8)		
14. Resisted finger abduction (T1)		
15. Babinski reflex test for UMN		

Continued

Upper Quarter Screening Exam	Normal	ABN
Lower Quarter Screening Exam*		
1. Postural assessment		
2. Active forward, backward, & lateral bending of lumbar spine		
3. Toe raises (S1)		
4. Heel walking (L4, L5)		
5. Active rotation of lumbar spine		
6. Overpressure if symptom-free		
7. Straight leg raise (L4, L5, S1)		
8. Sacroiliac spring test		
9. Resisted hip flexion (L1, L2)		
10. Passive ROM to hip		
11. Resisted knee extension (L3, L4)		
12. Knee flexion, extension, medial, & lateral tilt		
13. Femoral nerve stretch		
14. Babinski reflex test for UMN		

*Adapted from Cyriax & Cyriax: *Illustrated Manual of Orthop Med*, ed 2. Boston: Butterworth, 1993.

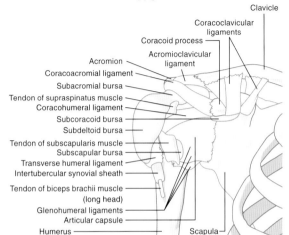

Shoulder joint anatomy: ligaments, bones, and bursa (R shoulder).

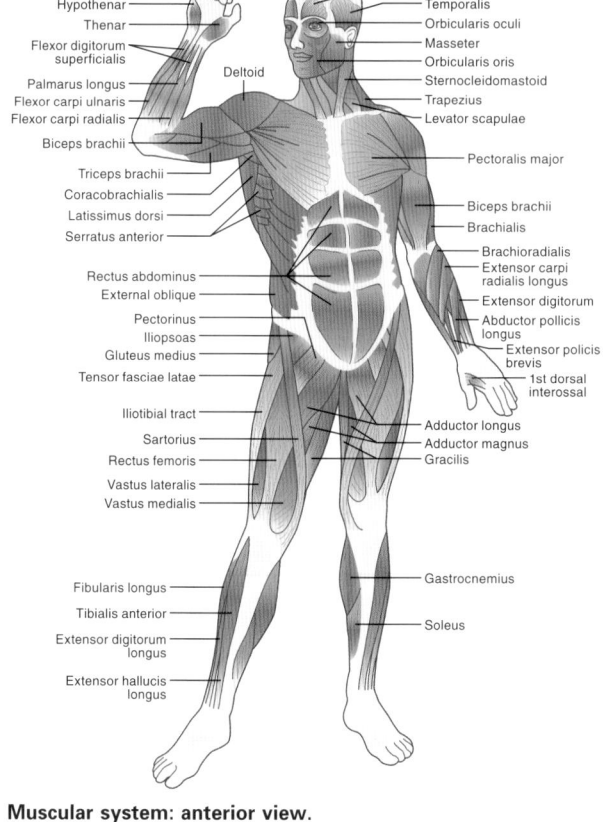

Muscular system: anterior view.

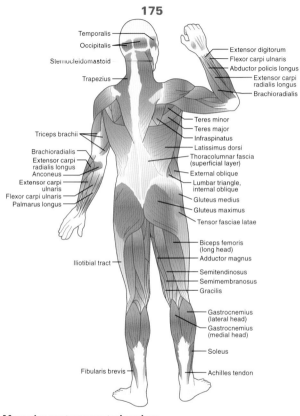

Temporalis
Occipitalis
Sternocleidomastoid
Trapezius

Extensor digitorum
Flexor carpi ulnaris
Abductor policis longus
Extensor carpi radialis longus
Brachioradialis

Teres minor
Teres major
Infraspinatus
Latissimus dorsi
Thoracolumnar fascia (superficial layer)
External oblique
Lumbar triangle, internal oblique
Gluteus medius
Gluteus maximus
Tensor fasciae latae

Triceps brachii
Brachioradialis
Extensor carpi radialis longus
Anconeus
Extensor carpi ulnaris
Flexor carpi ulnaris
Palmarus longus

Iliotibial tract

Biceps femoris (long head)
Adductor magnus
Semitendinosus
Semimembranosus
Gracilis

Gastrocnemius (lateral head)
Gastrocnemius (medial head)
Soleus

Fibularis brevis

Achilles tendon

Muscular system: posterior view.

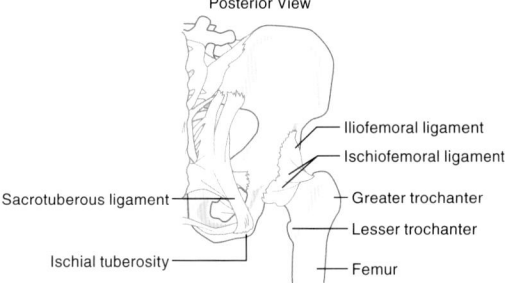

Anterior View

Anterior superior iliac spine
Inguinal ligament
Anterior inferior iliac spine
Iliopectineal bursa
Iliofemoral ligament
Greater trochanter
Intertrochanteric line
Lesser trochanter
Femur

Superior pubic ramus
Inferior pubic ramus
Obturator crest
Obturator foramen
Pubofemoral ligament

Posterior View

Sacrotuberous ligament

Ischial tuberosity

Iliofemoral ligament
Ischiofemoral ligament
Greater trochanter
Lesser trochanter
Femur

Hip joint anatomy: ligaments and bones.

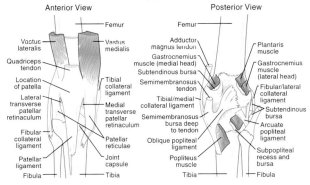

Knee joint anatomy: superficial ligaments and bones.

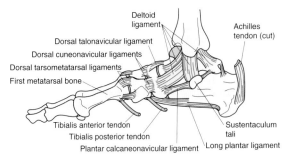

Ankle anatomy: Ligaments and bones.

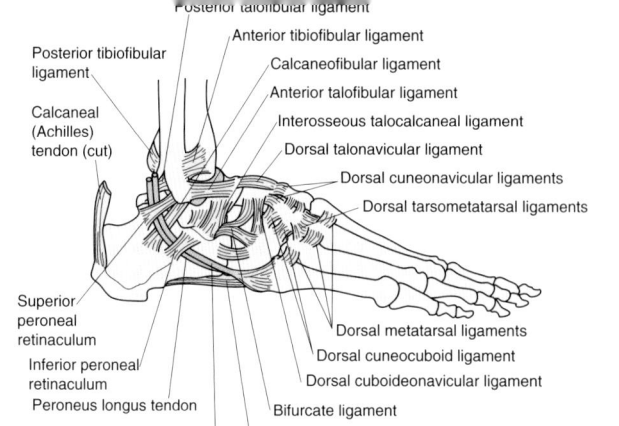

Posterior talofibular ligament

Anterior tibiofibular ligament

Posterior tibiofibular ligament

Calcaneofibular ligament

Anterior talofibular ligament

Calcaneal (Achilles) tendon (cut)

Interosseous talocalcaneal ligament

Dorsal talonavicular ligament

Dorsal cuneonavicular ligaments

Dorsal tarsometatarsal ligaments

Superior peroneal retinaculum

Dorsal metatarsal ligaments

Inferior peroneal retinaculum

Dorsal cuneocuboid ligament

Peroneus longus tendon

Dorsal cuboideonavicular ligament

Peroneus brevis tendon

Bifurcate ligament

Long plantar ligament

Ankle anatomy: Ligaments and bones.

Tests & Measures

Pain Assessment

Ransford Pain Assessment

Indicate location and type of pain. Use symbols to describe pain. Do not mark pain unrelated to present injury or condition.

///	Stabbing	x x x	Burning
000	Pins/Needles	= = =	Numbness

From Gulick D. *Ortho Notes*, ed. 2. Philadelphia: F.A. Davis, 2009. p.139.

Ransford Scoring System

The following are scored 2 pt each for pain in:	Points
Total leg	
Front of leg	
Anterior tibial	
Back of leg & knee	
Circumferential thigh	
Lateral whole leg	
Bilateral foot	
Circumferential foot	
Anterior knee & ankle	
Scattered throughout whole leg	
Entire abdomen	
Additional Points	
Drawings w/expansion or magnification of pain (1–2 pt) • Back pain radiating into iliac crest, groin, & anterior perineum • Pain drawn outside of diagram	
Additional explanations, circles, lines, arrows (1 pt each)	
Painful areas drawn in (1 pt for small area, 2 pt for large)	
Total Score	

Interpretation: A score of 3 or more points is thought to represent pain perception that may be influenced by psychological factors.

Pain Questions

1. Where is your pain?
2. What brings pain on?
3. What takes pain away?
4. Does pain travel to different areas?
5. Does pain always feel the same?
6. When is pain worst?
7. When is pain least?
8. Do you have joint swelling?

9. Do you have pain w/muscle spasms?
10. Do you have any numbness, tingling, burning pain?
11. Do you have hot or cold sensations with your pain?

Medical Screening for Possible Systemic Involvement: Associated Symptoms w/Pain

If "yes" to any of the following, check for presence of these Sx bilaterally (indicates referral to physician).

• Blumberg sign: rebound tenderness/pain on palpation • Burning • Difficulty breathing • Difficulty swallowing • Dizziness • Heart palpitations • Headache or visual changes • Hoarseness • Insidious onset w/no known mechanism of injury • Nausea • Numbness and/or tingling
No change in Sx despite positioning or rest
Night sweats
Pigmentation or changes, edema, rash, weakness, numbness, tingling, burning
Psoas test for pelvic pathology; SLR to 30° in supine & hip flex resisted
+ test for pelvic inflammation or infection/abdominal pain
− test indicates hip/back pain
Sx persist beyond expected healing time
Sx out of proportion to injury
Throbbing
Unexplained wt loss, pallor, bowel/bladder changes
Violent left shoulder pain (may be referred from spleen)
Vomiting
Weakness

Muscle Pain Referral Patterns

Supraspinatus.

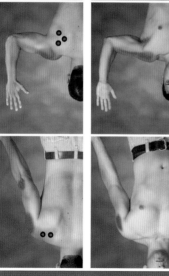

Infraspinatus.

Subscapularis.

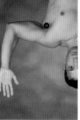

From Gulick D. *Ortho Notes*, ed. 2, p. 56–57.

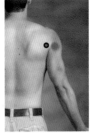 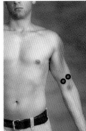

Teres minor.

Biceps brachii.

From Gulick D. *Ortho Notes,* ed. 2. p. 57.

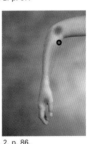 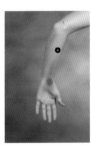

Brachioradialis.

Flexor carpi radialis.

From Gulick D. *Ortho Notes,* ed. 2. p. 86.

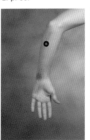 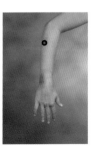

Flexor carpi ulnaris.

Extensor carpi ulnaris.

From Gulick D. *Ortho Notes,* ed. 2. pp. 86–87.

Extensor carpi radialis longus.

Extensor carpi radialis brevis.

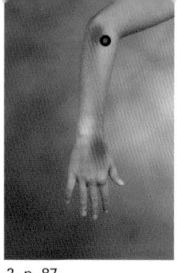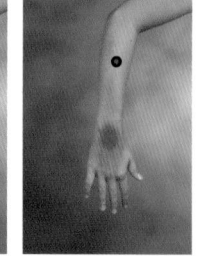

From Gulick D. *Ortho Notes,* ed. 2. p. 87.

Flexor digitorum.

Pronator teres.

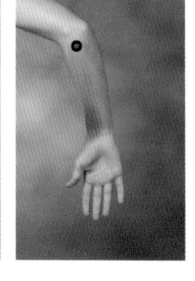

From Gulick D. *Ortho Notes,* ed. 2. p. 104.

Flexor pollicis longus.

First dorsal interossei.

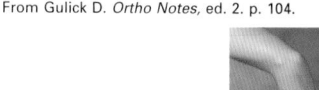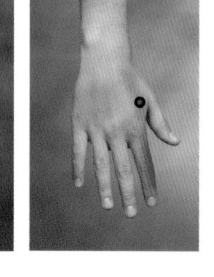

From Gulick D. *Ortho Notes,* ed. 2. p. 104.

185

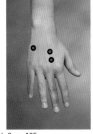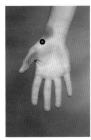

Abductor digiti minimi & second dorsal interossei.

Opponens pollicis.

From Gulick D. *Ortho Notes,* ed. 2. p. 105.

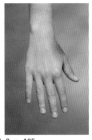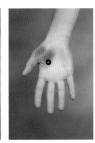

Adductor pollicis.

From Gulick D. *Ortho Notes,* ed. 2. p. 105.

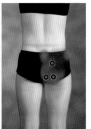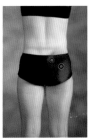

Gluteus maximus.

Piriformis.

From Gulick D. *Ortho Notes,* ed. 2. p. 188.

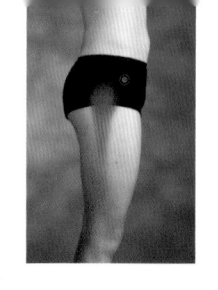

Tensor fascia latae.

From Gulick D. *Ortho Notes,* ed. 2. p. 188.

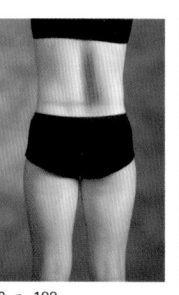 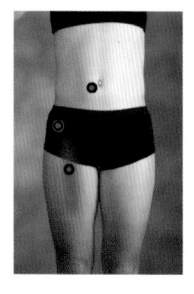

Iliopsoas.

From Gulick D. *Ortho Notes,* ed. 2. p. 188.

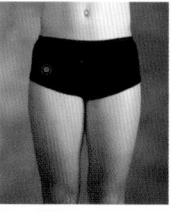 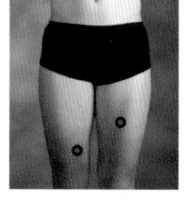

Rectus femoris.

Vasti muscles.

From Gulick D. *Ortho Notes,* ed. 2. p. 203.

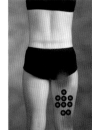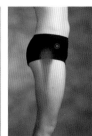

Hamstring muscles.

Tensor fascia latae.

From Gulick D. *Ortho Notes*, ed. 2. p. 204.

Range of Motion for Adults (AAOS)*

Joint/Motion	Range (in degrees)
Cervical spine—flexion	0–45
• extension	0–45
• lateral flexion	0–45
• rotation	0–60
Shoulder—flexion	0–180
• extension	0–60
• abduction	0–180
• internal rotation	0–70
• external rotation	0–90
• horizontal adduction	0–135
Elbow—flexion	0–150
Radioulnar—pronation	0–80
• supination	0–80
Wrist—flexion	0–80
• extension	0–70
• radial deviation	0–20
• ulnar deviation	0–30

Range of Motion for Adults (AAOS)—cont'd

Joint/Motion	Range (in degrees)
Thoracolumbar/lumbosacral—flexion	0–80 (or 4 in)
• extension	0–(20–30)
• lateral flex	0–35
• rotation	0–45
Hip—flexion	0–120
• extension	0–30
• abduction	0–45
• adduction	0–30
• internal rotation	0–45
• external rotation	0–45
Knee—flexion	0–135
Ankle—plantar flexion	0–50
• dorsiflexion	0–20
Subtalar—inversion	0–35
• eversion	0–15

*AAOS = American Academy of Orthopedic Surgeons.

Common End Feels w/Passive ROM

Capsular	Slow w/a building up of resistance (like stretching a belt; e.g., knee ext)
Ligamentous	Like capsular, but a little harder: solid stop w/o pain
Soft tissue approximation	Feels like a painful squeeze: movement stopped by contact w/adjacent soft tissue
Bone on bone	Hard, sudden stop
Muscle tightening/ elastic	Feel muscle reaction similar to other soft tissue, but hold-relax alters it: muscle tightness limits motion
Springlike	Muscle reaction is equal & opposite to pressure given, e.g., spring
Empty	Patient/client will not allow end feel due to pain

Common Capsular Patterns of Joints

Joint	Restriction
Temporamandibular	Limitation in mouth opening
Atlanto-occipital	Extension, side flexion equally limited
Cervical spine	Side flex & rotation equally limited, extension
Glenohumeral	Lateral rotation, abduction, medial rotation
Sternoclavicular	Pain at extreme ROM
Acromioclavicular	Pain at extreme ROM
Ulnohumeral	Flexion, extension
Radiohumeral	Flexion, extension, supination, pronation
Distal radioulnar	Full ROM, pain at extremes of rotation
Wrist	Flexion & extension equally limited
Trapeziometacarpal	Abduction, extension
Metacarpophalangeal or interphalangeal	Flexion, extension
Thoracic spine	Side flexion & rotation equally limited, extension
Lumbar spine	Side flexion & rotation equally limited, extension
Sacroiliac/symphysis pubis	Pain when joints stressed
Hip	Flexion, abduction, medial rotation
Knee	Flexion, extension
Talocrural	Plantar flexion, dorsiflexion
Subtalar	Limit of varus ROM
Midtarsal	Dorsiflexion, plantar flexion, adduction, medial rotation
First metatarsophalangeal	Flexion, extension

Adapted from Magee, D. *Orthopedic Physical Assessment*. St Louis: Saunders Elsevier; 2008. Table 1-16 p. 33.

Strength Assessment (muscle performance)

Grading System*

Grade	Definition
5 (NL)	Completes full ROM against gravity; maintains end-range against maximal resistance
4 (good)	Completes full ROM against gravity; maintains end-range against strong resistance
3+ (fair+)	Completes full ROM against gravity; maintains end-range against mild resistance
3 (fair)	Completes full ROM against gravity; unable to maintain end-range against any resistance
2 (poor)	Completes full ROM in a gravity-eliminated position
1 (trace)	Observable or palpated contractile activity in muscle w/o movement
0 (none)	No activity detected in muscle

*Hislop and Montgomery grading.

Optional Functional Muscle Testing for Lower Extremity

Chair Rise Test
Procedure: Participant sits on chair 43 cm in height with arms crossed in front of chest. Stand & sit down 5 times as fast as possible. Start timing on go & stop when returns to sit after 5th rise.
Normative data:
60–69: 11.4 sec
70–79: 12.6 sec
80–89: 12.7 sec

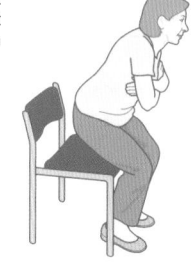

Bohannon 2006.

Thirty-Second Chair Rise

Procedure: Count number of times individual rises out of 43 cm ht chair without using arms & returns to sit.

Age	Norms Men	Norms Women
60–64	14–19	12–17
65–69	12–18	11–16
70–74	12–17	10–15
75–79	11–17	10–15
80–84	10–15	9–14
85–89	8–14	8–13
90–94	7–12	4–11

Visceral Innervation and Referral Patterns

Segmental Innervation	Viscera	Referral Pattern(s)
C3–5	Diaphragm	C-spine
T1–5	Heart	Anterior neck, chest, left UE
T4–6	Esophagus	Substernal & upper abdominal
T5–6	Lungs	T-spine
T6–10	Stomach	Upper abdomen & T-spine
	Pancreas	Upper abdomen, low T-spine, & upper L-spine
	Bile duct	Upper abdomen, mid T-spine
T7–9	Gallbladder	Right UQ, right T-spine
	Liver	Right T-spine
T7–10	Small intestine	Mid T-spine
T10–11	Testes/ovaries	Lower abdomen & sacrum
T10–L1	Kidney	L-spine, abdomen

Continued

Visceral Innervation and Referral Patterns—cont'd

Segmental Innervation	Viscera	Referral Pattern(s)
T10–L1 S2–4	Uterus Prostate	T/L & L/S junction Sacrum, testes, T/L jctn
T11–L2, S2–4	Ureter	Groin, suprapubic, medial thigh
	Bladder	Sacral apex, suprapubic

From Gulick D. *Ortho Notes,* ed. 2. p.4.

Joint Testing for Integrity and Nerve Involvement

Joint	Ligament/Joint Test	Description
Shoulder	Apprehension: anterior instability	Supine: abduct shoulder to 90° & ER to tolerance
	AC shear for AC sprain	AP compression of AC joint
	Coracoclavicular ligament test	Side-lying, UE behind back, abducted inferior angle of scapula (conoid) or abducted vertebral border of scapula (trapezoid)
	Neer: impingement of supraspinatus or biceps long head	Seated; passive movement of UE into full shoulder flex with humerus in IR
	Hawkins/Kennedy: impingement of supraspinatus	Seated; shoulder in 90° of flex and max IR
	Impingement relief test to confirm impingement	Seated; interior glide of GH joint, then elevate UE to full flex with humerus in Irqf

Joint Testing for Integrity and Nerve Involvement—cont'd

Joint	Ligament/Joint Test	Description
Elbow	Medial & lateral collateral	Varus force = LCL/RCL Valgus force = MCL/UCL
	Pronator terest: median nerve entrapment	UE relaxed, supported, resist pronation of forearm
	Mill: lateral epicondylitis	UE relaxed, elbow extended passively, stretch wrist into flexion & pronation
	Passive test: medial epicondylitis	UE relaxed, elbow extended; stretch into wrist extension & supination
	Tinel: ulnar nerve	Elbow in flex, tap groove bet olecranon & medial epicondyle
Wrist & Hand	Collaterals of wrist & digits	Varus force = LCL/RCL Valgus force = MCL/UCL
	Finkelstein: deQuervain syndrome	Ulnarly deviate wrist w/hand in fist around thumb. + test = pain along EPB and APL
	Phalen: carpal tunnel syndrome (CTS)	Max flex wrists so dorsal surfaces of hands in full contact w/each other. Hold for 1 min
	Reverse Phalen (prayer sign): assess CTS	Max extend wrists so palms of hands in full contact w/each other. Hold for 1 min

Continued

Joint	Ligament/Joint Test	Description
Hip	Trendelenburg	Standing: on leg w/opposite limb raised: test is for weak gluteus medius if pelvis falls
	Scour	IR/ER hip w/abduction/adduction while applying compress force femur down to test for labral tear
	Thomas: hip flexor tightness	Supine with lumbar stabilized, involved LE extended. Flex contralateral hip to abdomen. Tight hip flexors if contralateral flexes
	Ely: tight rectus femoris	Side-lying or prone with hip in extension: flex knee
	Obert: tight ITB	Side-lying with involved hip up; extend involved hip & let LE drop into adduction. + if does not drop
	Piriformis	Supine or contralateral side-lying. Flex hip to 70°–80° with knee flex & apply downward force to make knee adduct (+ test when pain in buttocks or sciatic pain)
	Ant/post labral: assess for tear	Ant: supine w/hip in flex, ER & ABD; resist movement into extension, IR, add + if pain or click Post: supine w hip in flex, IR; add, resist movement into ext, ER & ABD
	Patrick (Faber): assess Hip/SI pathology	Supine: passively flex, abduct, & ER hip so that lat malleolus of involved is on knee of uninvolved LE. Apply pressure to flexed knee

Joint Testing for Integrity and Nerve Involvement—cont'd

Joint	Ligament/Joint Test	Description
Knee	Collaterals	Varus stress for LCL Valgus stress for MCL
	Lachman: assess for ACL laxity	Supine, knee flexed 30°, proximal tibia moved forward to test ACL. + if moves >5 mm
	Anterior drawer: assess for ACL laxity	Supine, foot on table, knee flexed to 80°–90°. Move proximal tibia forward on femur
	Posterior drawer	Supine, hip flexed 45°, knee flexed 90°, grasp back of proximal tibia, tibia drawn back on femur to test PCL
	Grind test (Zohler): chondromalacia	Supine, knee in extension, PT compresses quads superior to patella; resist patella movement
Ankle	Anterior drawer	Grasp postcalcaneus & move anterior on tibia/fibula to assess for ATF laxity
	Talar tilt: assess for laxity of ATF, CF, PTF	Apply varus stress on talus using calcaneus & plantar flexion to test ATF, in neutral (CF), & dorsiflexion (PTF)
	Squeeze: assess for syndesmotic sprain	Supine 2-knee extension; compress tibia/fibula together from proximal (at knee) distally to assess for syndesmotic sprain
	Thompson: assess for Achilles tendon tear	Prone; flex knee to 90° and squeeze mid 1/3 of calf. + if no plantar flexion
	Morton: for neuroma	In NWB grasp at transverse metatarsal arch, squeeze heads of metatarsals together. + if pain bet toe 2 & 3 or 4 & 5
	Bump: stress fracture	NWB, ankle in neutral; apply force with palm of hand to heel of patient/client's foot. + if pain at site of fracture
	Tinel: tibial nerve damage	NWB tap over posterior tibia just below and posterior to medial malleolus. + if paresthesias develop in foot

Adapted From Gulick D. *Ortho Notes*, ed. 2. Philadelphia: F.A. Davis, 2009. p.139.

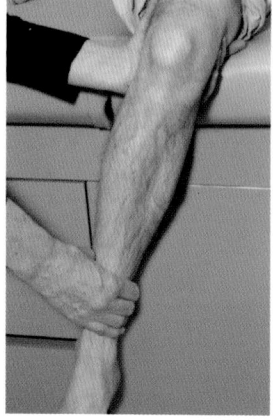

Valgus stress test.

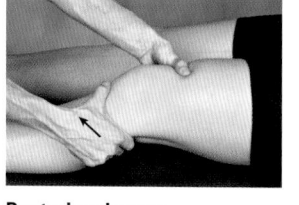

Posterior drawer.

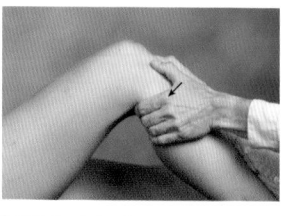

Lachman test.

From Gulick D. *Ortho Notes*, ed. 2. p. 204.

Assessment of Thoracic Outlet Syndrome

Testing for proximal compression of subclavian artery, vein, and/or brachial plexus involves placing patient/client in several positions that may provoke compression of these structures.

Method: Examiner monitors radial pulse of affected extremity.

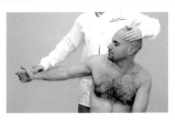

Response: Pulse rate slows: + test for compression of subclavian artery by anterior scalene muscle.

Method: Retract & depress shoulders from relaxed position: exaggerated military position.

Response: Onset of Sx or radial pulse slowing indicates + test for compression of neurovascular bundle.

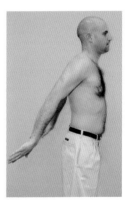

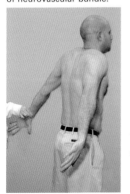

Method: Move affected arm(s) into abduction position: monitor pulse & Sx.

Response: Onset of Sx or radial pulse slowing.

Method: 3-min elevated arm test:
arms abducted to 90° & elbows
flexed to 90°; alternately, open &
close hands.
Response: + if unable to complete
3 min or onset of Sx.

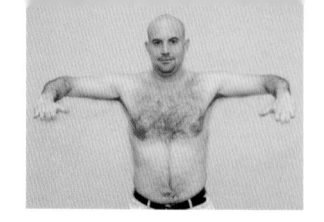

Spine Mobility Tests

Slump Test
To test for neural mobility.
Position: Patient/client seated with
trunk in slumped posture while
maintain neck flex.
Method: Add knee extension of one
LE w/dorsiflexion, & then repeat
with other LE.

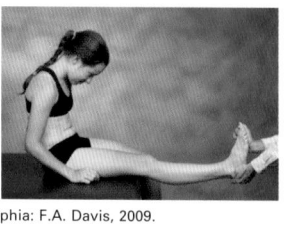

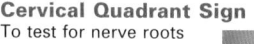
From Gulick D. *Ortho Notes*, ed. 2. Philadelphia: F.A. Davis, 2009.

Cervical Quadrant Sign
To test for nerve roots
and IVF
Position: Patient/client
seated.
Method: Stand behind
with fingers interlocked
on top of head,
compress w/C-spine in
slight extension &
lateral flex.

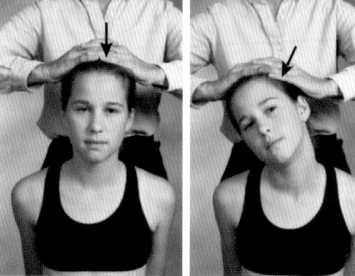

From Gulick D. *Ortho Notes*, ed. 2. Philadelphia: F.A. Davis, 2009.

Cervical Distraction Test

To assess nerve root impingement & cervical mobility.
Position: Patient/client supine or seated.
Method: Impart controlled distraction force of C-spine to decompress facet jts.

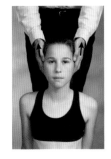

From Gulick D. *Ortho Notes*, ed. 2. Philadelphia: F.A. Davis, 2009.

Vertebral Artery Test

To assess integrity of int carotid arteries.
Position: Patient/client supine.
Method: Hands under occiput; extend & side bend C-spine & rotate 45° & hold for 30 sec.

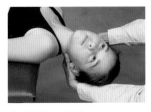

From Gulick D. *Ortho Notes*, ed. 2. Philadelphia: F.A. Davis, 2009.

Transverse Ligament

Position: Patient/client supine, head cradled in tester's hands. Stabilize C2 arches with thumbs.
Method: Lift occiput w/cupped hands & translate head forward. Hold 15 sec.

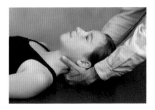

From Gulick D. *Ortho Notes*, ed. 2. Philadelphia: F.A. Davis, 2009.

Lateral A & P Rib

To assess for fracture.

Position: Patient/client supine.

Method: On lateral aspect of rib cage compress bilaterally, then put hands on front & back of chest.

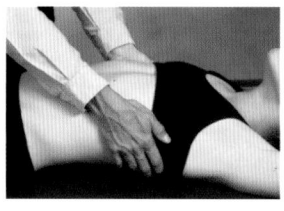 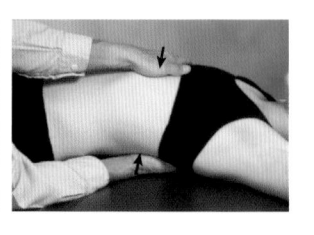

From Gulick D. *Ortho Notes*, ed. 2. Philadelphia: F.A. Davis, 2009.

Beevor Sign

To assess abdominal musculature.

Position: Patient/client supine w/knees flexed & feet on mat.

Method: Head & shoulders raised off mat while umbilicus is observed (should remain in straight line).

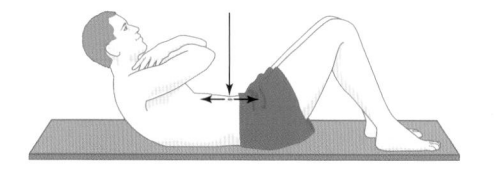

SLR Test
Position: Patient/client supine hip flex, adduct, IR, & knee extended.
Method:

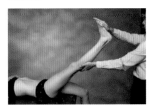

A. Dorsiflex: looking at sciatic.

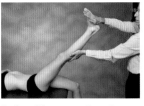

B. Dorsiflex, eversion, & toe extension: tibial.

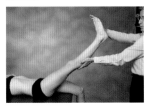

C. Dorsiflex and inversion: sural.

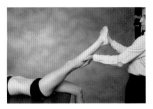

D. Plantarflex and invert: common perineal.

From Gulick D. *Ortho Notes*, ed. 2. Philadelphia: F.A. Davis, 2009.

SI Posterior Compression
Position: Patient/client supine.
Method: Clinician's hands crossed over pelvis on ASIS; apply lateral force to ASIS through hands.

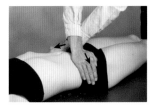

From Gulick D. *Ortho Notes*, ed. 2. Philadelphia: F.A. Davis, 2009.

SI Posterior Gapping Test
SI Posterior Gapping Test
Position: Patient/client side-lying.
Method: Apply a downward force
through ant aspect of ASIS to
create posterior gapping of SI.

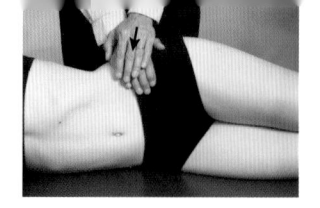

Hoover Test
To assess malingering.
Position: Patient/client supine.
Method: Hold patient/client's heels
of bilat leg in clinician's hands.
Ask patient/client to lift one leg out
of hand (positive if patient/client
does not lift leg, & no force being
applied).

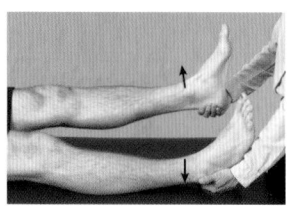

From Gulick D. *Ortho Notes*, ed. 2. Philadelphia: F.A. Davis, 2009.

Spinal Mobility

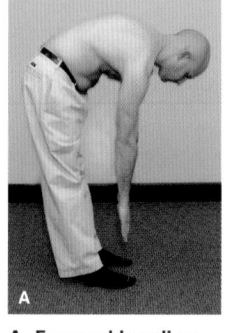

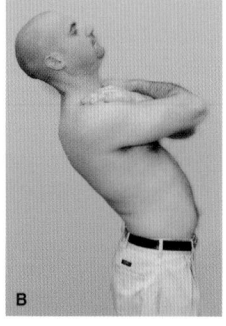

**A. Forward bending
motion. Facets open.**

**B. Backward bending
motion. Facets closed.**

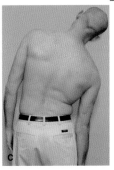

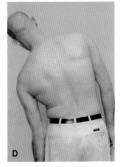

C. Side bending right motion. Right facet closes, left facet opens.

D. Side bending left motion. Right facet opens, left facet closes.

Spine Medical Red Flags

- Individuals <20 and >55 y with persistent night pain, change in bowel & bladder, bilateral LE signs, PMH of Ca, nonechanical pain, SED >25
- Mid-thoracic pain = MI or GB
- Pain from 6th–10th thoracic vertebra = peptic ulcer
- History of prostate CA
- Pulsing LBP = vascular problem (aortic aneurysm?)
- Fraun beard = spina bifida
- Café au lait spots = neurofibromatosis
- Upper back/neck pain that ↑ w/deep breathing, coughing, laughing, & ↓ with breath hold; recent Hx may include fever, URI, flu, MI, or pericarditis
- Enlarged cervical lymph nodes, severe pruritus, irregular fever = Hodgkin disease
- Pain at McBurney point = 1/2 the distance from ASIS to umbilicus; tenderness = appendicitis

Gulick, 2009.

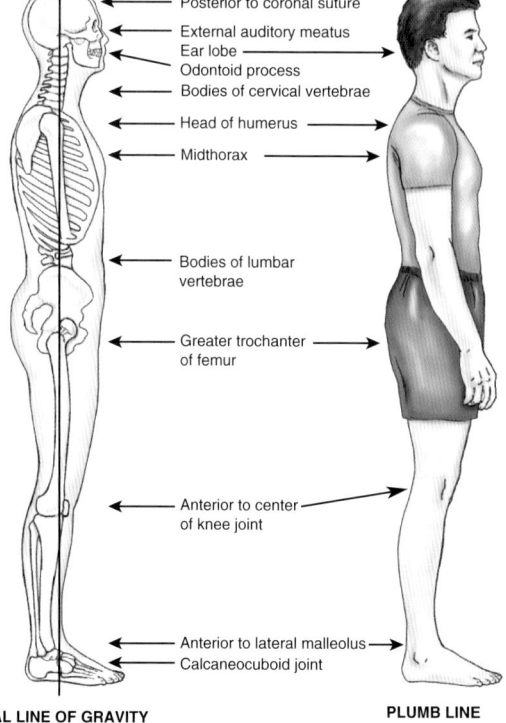

ANATOMIC LANDMARKS

SURFACE LANDMARKS

Posterior to coronal suture

External auditory meatus
Ear lobe
Odontoid process
Bodies of cervical vertebrae

Head of humerus

Midthorax

Bodies of lumbar
vertebrae

Greater trochanter
of femur

Anterior to center
of knee joint

Anterior to lateral malleolus
Calcaneocuboid joint

IDEAL LINE OF GRAVITY

PLUMB LINE

Posture Assessment *(continued)*

ANATOMIC LANDMARKS

SURFACE LANDMARKS

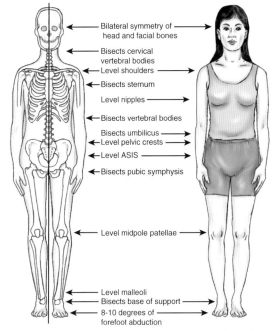

- Bilateral symmetry of head and facial bones
- Bisects cervical vertebral bodies
- Level shoulders
- Bisects sternum
- Level nipples
- Bisects vertebral bodies
- Bisects umbilicus
- Level pelvic crests
- Level ASIS
- Bisects pubic symphysis
- Level midpole patellae
- Level malleoli
- Bisects base of support
- 8-10 degrees of forefoot abduction

IDEAL LINE OF GRAVITY

PLUMB LINE

Risk Factors for Chronicity of Spinal Dysfunction

Physical Factors	Psychological/Legal/Occupational
• Smoker • Numbness & paresthesia in same distribution • Radiating LE pain • Previous LBP • Poor fitness	• Total work loss secondary LBP • Adversarial legal proceedings • Low job satisfaction • Depression • Personal problems: alcohol, marital, financial

Postural Variations

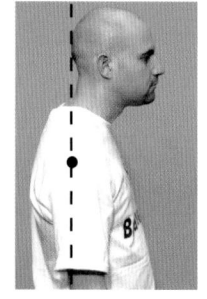

Forward head.

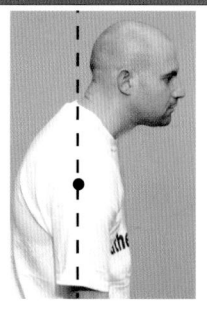

Kyphosis.

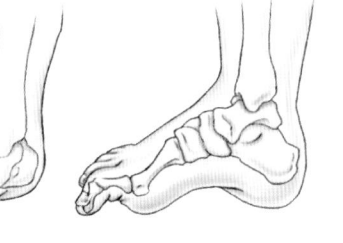

Pronated foot.

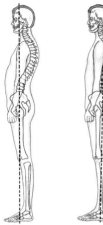 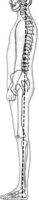 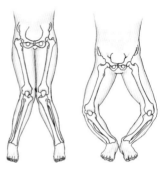

Increased lordosis.   **Flat back.**   **A. Genu valgus. B. Genu varus.**

Motor Control				
Task Level of Impairment				
	Intact	**Min**	**Mod**	**Max**
Perception				
Attention				
Cognition				
Arousal				
Sensation				
Tone				

Continued

Motor Control—cont'd

Task Level of Impairment

	Intact	Min	Mod	Max
Mov't patterns				
Sitting balance				
Standing balance				

Courtesy of Dawn Gulick.

Postural Deformities

Deformity	Common Problems Associated w/Deformity
Forward head position	Upper cervical pain, headache; progresses to spinal deformities: e.g., thoracic kyphosis, & ↓ lumbar lordosis
Cervical/thoracic kyphosis	Upper cervical pain, headache, abducted scapulae, stretched & weak posterior trunk muscles, shortened anterior musculature
Scapular winging Scapular elevation/ depression Scapular retraction	Weak UEs, weak scapular stabilizers (serratus, mid & lower trapezius) Muscle spasms in upper thoracic area
↑ lumbar lordosis	Hypermobile in extension, hypomobile in flexion, sheer stresses to L4, L5 & L5, S1; ↓ strength of abdominal muscles, shortened hip flexors: ↑ risk of disk disease
↓ lumbar lordosis	May lead to disk disease
Genu valgus (a) Genu varus (b)	(a) Leads to medial knee & ankle pain & lateral hip pain. (b) Lateral knee & ankle pain
Pes planus (flat foot)	↑ Valgus stress on knees; ABN stress on joints of foot
Pes cavus (high arch)	↑ Stress on all LE structures & spine

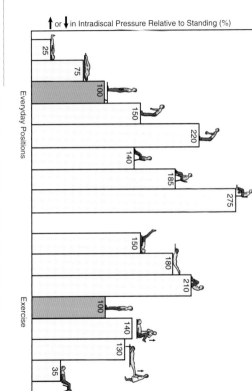

↑ or ↓ in Intradiscal Pressure Relative to Standing (%)

Everyday Positions

25
75
100
150
220
140
185
275

Exercise

150
180
210
100
140
130
35

Ergonomics & Body Mechanics

From Nachemson A. The lumbar spine: An orthopedic challenge. *Spine* 1:50–71, 1976.

Prevention of Neck & Back Injuries

Activities: Sleeping.
Correct Positions: Pillow should keep spine straight, & neck & lumbar back in neutral.

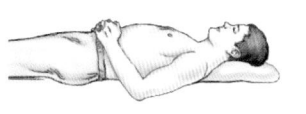 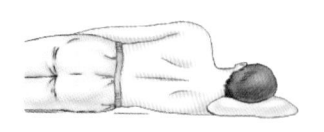

Activities: Sitting at work.
Correct Positions: Desk, chair, & monitor adjusted so monitor is eye level.
Use armrest.
Sit w/spine against back of chair.
Knees slightly lower than hips.
Use footstool.
Correct Positions: Move fingers only.
Maintain a straight-wrist position.
Consider wrist splints to decrease work on wrists.

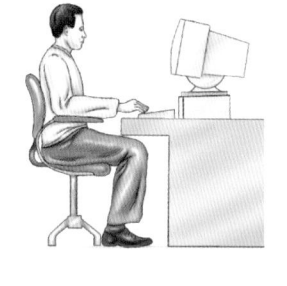

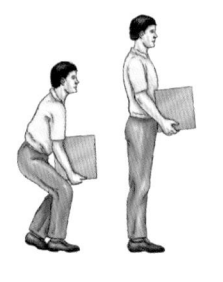

Activities: Lifting heavy objects.
Correct Positions: Keep object close to your center of gravity.
Contract abdominals.
Use legs & hips to lift, not neck & back.

Gait, Locomotion, & Balance

Observational Gait Analysis	NL	ABN
Reciprocal arm swing		
Rotation of shoulders & thorax		
Pelvic rotation		
Hip flexion & extension (min flexion: 30°)		
Knee flexion & extension (min flexion: 40°; 70° for stairs)		
Ankle dorsiflexion & plantar flexion (min 15° dorsiflexion, 15° plantar flexion)		
Step length (right = left)		
Stride length (NL = 70–82 cm or 27–32 in)		
Heel rise		
Pre-swing		
Cadence (NL = 90–120 steps/min)		
Pelvic rotation		
Pelvic list		
Hip rotation & abduction/adduction		
Knee rotation & abduction/adduction		
Degree of toeing-out		
Base of support measurement		
Subtalar movement		

Abnormalities of Gait

Phase	Deviations	Causes/Problems
Both	Antalgic gait: • Decrease in duration of stance of affected limb • Lack of wt shift over stance limb • Decrease in swing phase of uninvolved side	Pain in lower limb or pelvic region Limited ROM or strength in 1 extremity
Both	Trendelenburg gait: Pelvis drops on unaffected side during single-limb support of side of weakness, or lurching gait w/laterally flexing of trunk over affected limb	Gluteus medius weakness
Stance: heel strike	Quick moving of trunk posteriorly at initial contact w/ground, allowing for upright posture to be maintained	Paralysis or weakness of gluteus maximus
Stance	When shorter limb makes contact w/ground: pelvis drops laterally, longer limb joints show exaggerated flexion or circumduction	Leg length discrepancy
	Lengthening of uninvolved limb (hip hiking) to achieve swing-through of affected limb	Joint hypomobility of hip or knee flexion
	Forward bending of trunk w/rapid plantar flexion to create extension	Inability of quadriceps to contract
Stance	Diminished stance phase of affected side & smaller step length on unaffected side; no true propulsion because of weakness	Weakness or paralysis of ankle plantar flexors
	Increased lumbar lordosis & backward bending of trunk	Hip flexion contracture
	Early heel rise during terminal stance; knee hyperextension at midstance & forward bending of trunk w/hip flexion	Plantar flexion contracture

Abnormalities of Gait—cont'd

Phase	Deviations	Causes/Problems
Swing	Difficulty in initiating swing-through; rotates limb externally at hip, using adductors to achieve swing-through	Weakness of psoas muscle
	Steppage gait; increased hip & knee flexion to compensate for dropfoot	Lack of ankle dorsiflexion
	Foot slap during ground contact	Weak anterior tibialis
	Excessive dorsiflexion of ankle during late swing phase to early stance of uninvolved limb; involved limb: early heel rise in terminal stance	Knee flexion contracture

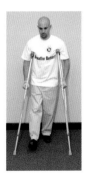

Gait Training w/Assistive Devices

Gait Pattern: Three-point pattern using unilateral assistive device.

Description: Assistive device on opposite side of involved lower limb. Start: assistive device advanced, involved lower limb, then uninvolved lower limb. Walker forward first, then involved limb, then uninvolved limb.

Gait Pattern: Four-point pattern for bilateral assistive device.

Description: One crutch, contralateral lower limb, other crutch, then other lower limb.

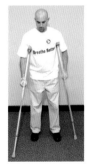

Gait Pattern: Two point pattern: assistive device & involved lower limb move together.
Description: Assistive device & involved lower limb move forward, then uninvolved lower limb. Walker forward first, non-weight-bearing involved limb forward, then uninvolved limb.

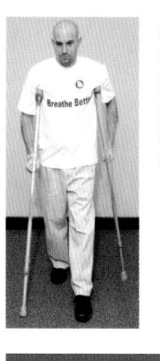

Gait Pattern: Stair climbing.
Description: Ascend stairs w/ uninvolved leg first, followed by involved leg & assistive device. Descend stairs w/assistive device & involved leg first, then uninvolved leg.

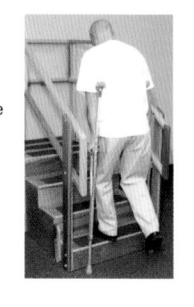

Self-Care & Home Management Assessment

Level of Assistance Required					
Task	Independent	Supervised	Min	Mod	Max
Bed mobility: roll side to side	I	S	Min	Mod	Max
Move up & down in bed	I	S	Min	Mod	Max
Supine to sit/sit to supine	I	S	Min	Mod	Max
WC mobility; propel on straight surfaces	I	S	Min	Mod	Max
Propel around cones & through doors	I	S	Min	Mod	Max
Endurance for community	I	S	Min	Mod	Max
Transfers: sit/stand & stand/sit	I	S	Min	Mod	Max

Level of Assistance Required					
Task	Independent	Supervised	Min	Mod	Max
WC/stand to low bed or toilet	I	S	Min	Mod	Max
WC/stand to floor	I	S	Min	Mod	Max
WC/stand to bathtub	I	S	Min	Mod	Max
WC/stand to car	I	S	Min	Mod	Max
Gait activities: level surfaces	I	S	Min	Mod	Max
Ascends stairs	I	S	Min	Mod	Max
Descends stairs	I	S	Min	Mod	Max
Ramps	I	S	Min	Mod	Max
Endurance for community activities	I	S	Min	Mod	Max
ADL assessment: bathing	I	S	Min	Mod	Max
Toileting	I	S	Min	Mod	Max
Dressing	I	S	Min	Mod	Max
Cooking	I	S	Min	Mod	Max

MS Diagnostics

Diagnostic Test: X-ray
Indications: Initial test to evaluate what can't be seen by observation; evaluate abnormalities from palpation
Info Gathered: Tumor, fracture, vascular abnormality, soft tissue abnormality, etc
Precautions/Notes: Pregnancy
Diagnostic Test: CT
Indications: To detect more info about any part of body
Info Gathered: Detailed visualization of parts scanned; location of tumors, tears, etc
Precautions/Notes: Check for allergy to contrast (if contrast given); claustrophobia
Diagnostic Test: MRI
Indications: Detect changes in tissue not seen on CT or X-ray

Info Gathered: Changes in joints, ligaments, & cartilage; bone infection, disease, tumor, fracture; spine: disk herniation

Precautions/Notes: Check for claustrophobia; metal implants (those containing iron are contraindicated); pacemaker, artificial limbs, etc; if female has IUD; if contrast being used (patient/client may have allergy to contrast)

Diagnostic Test: Radionuclide scintigraphy (bone scan)

Indications: Hot spot imaging to detect areas of fracture, NL or ABN fracture healing, metastatic bone tumors, benign tumors, Paget disease, AVN, osteomyelitis

Info Gathered: Reveals early bone disease or bone healing

Precautions/Notes: Not specific in differential diagnosis; must be used w/other lab, imaging, & clinical tests

Diagnostic Test: Dual energy X-ray; absorptiometry

Indications: To evaluate bone mineral density: usually lower spine & hip areas evaluated

Info Gathered: Amount of Ca^{++} in certain regions of bones; estimation of bone strength; estimation of risk for fracture

Precautions/Notes: No known risks or side effects

MS Interventions

<table>
<tr><td colspan="2" align="center">More Common Orthotic, Protective,
& Supportive Devices</td></tr>
<tr><td>Orthotic Defined by Location</td><td align="center">Description/Indication</td></tr>
<tr><td colspan="2">Cervical</td></tr>
<tr><td>1. Soft foam/rubber collar
2. Philadelphia collar
3. SOMI
4. Halo</td><td>1. Support the neck; ↓ work of neck muscles; minimal motion control
2. Rigid plastic supports chin & posterior head: greater motion control
3. Major restriction of all motion at neck w/4 posts
4. Total restriction/maximal orthotic control: circular band of metal fixed to skull by 4 screws</td></tr>
</table>

More Common Orthotic, Protective, & Supportive Devices—cont'd

Orthotic Defined by Location	Description/Indication
Back	
1. Lumbosacral orthosis (Knight spinal) 2. Thoracolum-bosacral (Taylor brace)	1. Rigid trunk orthosis w/a pelvic & thoracic band & posterior uprights; restrains flexibility, controls extension, & limits lateral flexibility 2. Pelvic band & posterior uprights to midscapular level; reduces flexibility, lateral flexibility, & extension; limits trunk motion
Shoulder	
1. Acromioclavicular separation splint 2. Hemiplegia sling	1. For mgmt of an AC separation or postsurgery 2. Used post CVA to prevent trauma to AC joint & GH subluxation
Wrist	
1. Static resting splint 2. Carpal tunnel splints	1. Maintains wrist joint in ext w/mild pressure to surface of hand: assists w/ healing postsurgery or postinjury; may or may not splint each finger 2. Maintains wrist in neutral to prevent pressure on median nerve
Knee	
1. Cho-Pat 2. Controlled motion knee brace 3. Palumbo patellar stabiliza-tion brace	1. Rubber strap placed at site of patellofemoral tendon 2. & 3. To protect area of injury, delimit extent of swelling & tissue damage, & control patient/client knee pain; also used to limit motion in sports activities for months after knee surgery
Ankle-Foot Orthosis	Plastic or metal orthoses used to compensate for paralysis of entire leg & provide dorsiflexion assistance; used in stroke, peripheral neuropathy, incomplete spinal cord injury

Conditions Requiring Special Precautions During Transfers

Conditions	Special Precautions
Total hip replacement, especially within first 2 weeks after surgery	• Prevent hip adduction, internal rotation, & flexion >90° • No hip extension beyond neutral flexion-extension • Use a raised toilet seat & chair
Low back trauma or discomfort	• Avoid excessive lumbar rotation, side & forward bend • Teach log rolling • Hips & knees should be partially flexed when in supine or side-lying

Salter Fracture Classification

Descriptors of Fracture	Definition
Site: Diaphyseal (a) Metaphyseal (b) Epiphyseal (c) Intra-articular (d)	(a) Shaft (b) Conical portion between shaft & epiphysis of long bone (c) Center of bone growth at articular end of bone (d) W/in the joint
Extent: Complete or incomplete	If incomplete: can be crack, hairline, buckle, or green-stick fracture
Configuration: Transverse oblique/spiral/comminuted	Complete fractures defined as crosswise across long axis (transverse), slanting (oblique), or spiral (coiled, winding around the long axis); more than 2 fragments (comminuted)
Relationship of fracture fragments: Displaced vs. nondisplaced	If displaced: can be shifted sideways, angulated, rotated, distracted, overriding, or impacted

Salter Fracture Classification—cont'd

Descriptors of Fracture	Definition
Relationship to external environment: Closed (simple) vs. open (compound)	Closed: skin intact Open: skin in area not intact
Complications: Complicated vs. uncomplicated	Complicated has either local or systemic complication; increases healing time

Types of Fractures

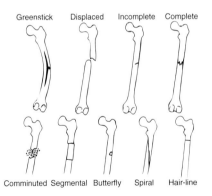

From Rothstein RM, Roy SH, Wolf SL. *The Rehabilitation Specialist's Handbook*, FA Davis: Philadelphia; 2005; ed.3. p. 84.

Special Considerations/Populations & Differential Diagnosis

Effect of Immobilization

Examples of Immobilization: Cast, Bedrest, Weightlessness, Denervation (SCI or Nerve Injury), Self-Imposed Due to Pain, Inflammation

Types of Tissue	Adaptation to ↓ Load	Result	Time for Change	Recovery
Ligament/ tendon	↓ collagen content ↓ cross-linking ↓ tensile strength	Weakening of tissue	↓ tensile strength & stiffness by 50% after 8 wk	12–18 mo
Articular surface (joint, menisci, underlying bone)	↓ proteoglycan content ↓ collagen synthesis Cartilage atrophy Regional osteoporosis ↓ strength of ligaments at insertion sites ↑ H$_2$O content of cartilage	↓ ROM available to joint ↓ time from load to failure ↓ energy-absorbing capacity of bone-ligament complex Weakening of muscle around joint	Unknown	Unknown
Cartilage	Thinning of cartilage Advancing of subchondral bone	↓ ROM due to ↑ bone	Unknown	Unknown

Effect of Immobilization—cont'd

Examples of Immobilization: Cast, Bedrest, Weightlessness, Denervation (SCI or Nerve Injury), Self-Imposed Due to Pain, Inflammation

Types of Tissue	Adaptation to ↓ Load	Result	Time for Change	Recovery
Joint capsule	Disordered collagen fibrils AB cross-linking	Capsular stiffness, ↓ joint mobility	Unknown	Unknown
Synovium	Adhesion formation Fibro-fatty tissue proliferation into joint space	↓ gliding, ↓ fluid movement	Unknown	Unknown
Muscle	Muscle atrophy: • Atrophy of type I fibers • If CNS damage: atrophy of type II fibers Joint contractures cause limits in ROM Alternate patterns of movement Vascular & fluid stasis	Within 3 d of immobilization	For every d of immobilization, may take up to 2 d of strengthening to return to NL strength	

Fibromyalgia Screening

1. Do you have trouble sleeping through the night?	Yes	No
2. Do you feel rested in the morning?	Yes	No
3. Are you stiff & sore in the morning?	Yes	No
4. Do you have daytime fatigue/exhaustion?	Yes	No
5. Does your muscle pain & soreness travel to different places on your body?	Yes	No
6. Do you have tension/migraine headaches?	Yes	No
7. Do you have irritable bowel Sx (nausea, diarrhea, cramping)?	Yes	No
8. Do you have swelling, numbness, or tingling in your arms/legs?	Yes	No
9. Are you sensitive to temperature & humidity or changes in the weather?	Yes	No
Total:		

Scoring: If yes to 2 or more questions, patient/client may have fibromyalgia.

Fibromyalgia tender points: >11 out of 18 is positive diagnosis.

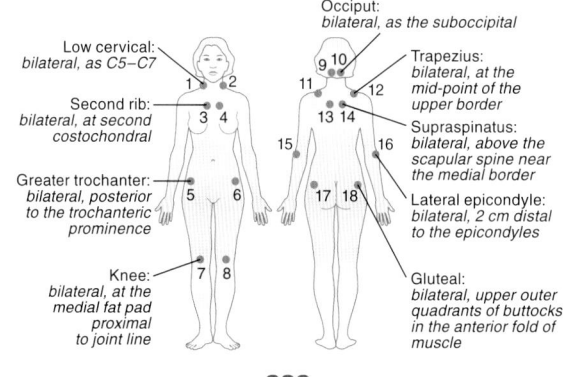

Occiput:
bilateral, as the suboccipital

Low cervical:
bilateral, as C5–C7

Trapezius:
bilateral, at the mid-point of the upper border

Second rib:
bilateral, at second costochondral

Supraspinatus:
bilateral, above the scapular spine near the medial border

Greater trochanter:
bilateral, posterior to the trochanteric prominence

Lateral epicondyle:
bilateral, 2 cm distal to the epicondyles

Knee:
bilateral, at the medial fat pad proximal to joint line

Gluteal:
bilateral, upper outer quadrants of buttocks in the anterior fold of muscle

222

Osteoporosis Screening Evaluation

Evaluation Questions	Yes	No
1. Do you have a small, thin body?		
2. Are you white or Asian?		
3. Have any of your blood-related family members had osteoporosis?		
4. Are you a postmenopausal woman?		
5. Do you drink ≥2 oz of alcohol each day? (1 beer, 1 glass wine or 1 cocktail = 1 oz alcohol)		
6. Do you smoke more than 10 cigarettes each day?		
7. Are you physically active? (walk or similar exercise 3 ×/week)		
8. Have you had both ovaries removed before age 40 y w/o hormone replacement?		
9. Have you been taking thyroid, anti-inflammatory, or seizure medications >6 mo?		
10. Have you broken your hip, spine, or wrist?		
11. Do you drink or eat >3 servings of caffeine, tea, coffee, or chocolate/day?		
12. Is your diet low in dairy products or other sources of calcium?		
If you answer yes to 3 or more questions, you may be at greater risk for developing osteoporosis		

Comparison of Osteoarthritis & Rheumatoid Arthritis

Characteristics	OA	RA
Age of onset	Usually >40 y	Usually >15 & <50 y
Progression	Develops slowly over many y due to mechanical stress	May develop suddenly in wk/mo

Continued

Comparison of Osteoarthritis & Rheumatoid Arthritis—cont'd

Characteristics	OA	RA
Manifestations	Osteophyte formation, cartilage destruction, altered joint alignment	Inflammatory synovitis, irreversible structural damage to joint & bone
Joint involvement	Few joints: DIP, PIP, first CMC of hands Cervical & lumbar spine Hips, knees, & first MTP of foot	Many joints, bilaterally MCP, PIP, hands, wrists, elbows, shoulders, cervical spine MTP, ankle
Joint S & S	Morning stiffness (>30 min) ↑ joint pain w/ weight-bearing joints & activity	Redness, warmth, swelling, prolonged morning stiffness
Systemic S & S	Weight-bearing joints Asymmetrical involvement	General feeling of sickness, fatigue Wt loss, fever, rheumatoid nodules Ocular, hematological, & cardiac Sx Non-weight-bearing joints Symmetrical involvement

Amputee & Prosthetic Management

Clinical concerns when evaluating potential for prostheses

- Cognitive dysfunction that interferes w/training
- Advanced neurological disorders
- Cardiopulmonary conditions severe enough to impose limitations on effort
- Ulcers or infections with compromised circulation
- Irreducible and pronounced knee flexion contractures in below-knee candidates and hip flexion contractures in above-knee candidates

Other factors to consider

- Older age
- Multiple comorbidities (especially diabetes and/or PAD)
- Psychosocial factors (diminished body image, level of emotional readiness, or presence of depression or decreased quality of life)

Guccione, 2012.

Levels for Prosthesis Use & Commonly Prescribed Prostheses for the Older Adult

	Functional Level	Amputee Mobility Predictor Score
K0	Does not have ability to ambulate or transfer safely w/ or w/out assistance; prosthesis does not enhance quality of life	<9.67
K1	Has ability to use prosthesis for amb on level surface at fixed cadence; typical of limited & **unlimited household ambulator** Suspension: hip control w/pelvic belt, silesian belt, gel locking liner, or lanyard for transfemoral, supracondylar, or patella tendon bearing suction on a case by case basis Socket: ischial containment for transfemoral; patella tendon bearing total contact for transtibial Socket inserts: locking or cushion gel liners (2 per prosthesis) Knee: single axis, constant friction, stance phase lock, manual locking, or polycentric Ankle/foot: SACH or single axis	>9.6 / Avg. 25
K2	Has the ability/potential for ambulation w/ability to transverse low-level environmental barriers, curbs, stairs, uneven surfaces. **Limited community ambulator** Suspension: same as K1; suction considered Socket & knee: Same as K1 Ankle/foot: flexible-keel foot or multiaxial foot, axial rotation unit, dynamic prosthetic pylon Mobility predictor score >25.28	>25.28 Avg. 34.65

Continued

	Functional Level	Amputee Mobility Predictor Score
K3	Has the ability/potential for ambulation w/variable cadence; has ability to traverse most environmental barriers & may have vocational, therapeutic, or exercise activity demanding prosthetic utilization beyond simple locomotion: typical of the **community ambulator**	>31.96 Avg. 40.5
K4	Has ability/potential for prosthetic ambulation that exceeds basic amb skills; exhibits high impact, stress, or energy levels; **typical of prosthetic demands of child, active adult, or athlete** Suspension: same as K1 Socket: Same as K1 Knee: fluid, pneumatic, or computerized knee Ankle/foot: flex foot or flex-walk system; energy storing foot, multiaxial ankle/foot, dynamic response, shank/foot system w/vertical loading pylon	>38.49 Avg. 44.67

AMPPRO and AMPnoPRO assess functional potential for unilateral amputee w/ and w/o prosthesis. Bilateral use AMPPRO only. Total range for AMPPRO is 0–42. Total for AMPnoPRO is 38.

Gait Deviations in Prosthetics

Observational gait

- Deviations observed
- ( ) No significant deviations observed
- ( ) Trunk lateral lean
- ( ) Forward trunk flexion
- ( ) Hip hiking
- ( ) Hip circumduction
- ( ) Scissoring
- ( ) Trendelenburg R ___L___

- ( ) Knee hyperextension R __L__
- ( ) Foot drop R ___L___
- ( ) Ataxic gait pattern
- ( ) Antalgic gait pattern
- ( ) Festinating
- ( ) Shuffling
- ( ) Decreased gait speed
- ( ) Widened base of support
- ( ) OTHER:

PNF UE Diagonal Patterns

I. UE Diagonal Patterns

A. D1 flexion

Scapula-anterior elevation
Shoulder-flexion, adduction, ER
Elbow-varies
Forearm-supination
Wrist-radial flexion
Fingers-radial flexion
Thumb- flexion, adduction

B. D1 extension

Scapula-posterior depression
Shoulder-extension, abduction, IR
Elbow-varies
Forearm-pronation
Wrist-ulnar extension
Fingers-ulnar extension
Thumb- extension, abduction

C. D2 flexion

Scapula-posterior elevation
Shoulder-flexion, abduction, ER
Elbow-varies
Forearm-supination
Wrist-radial extension
Fingers-radial extension
Thumb- extension, abduction

D. D2 extension

Scapula-anterior depression
Shoulder-extension, adduction, IR
Elbow-varies
Forearm-pronation
Wrist-ulnar flexion
Fingers-ulnar flexion
Thumb- flexion, opposition

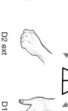

D1 flex

D2 flex

D2 ext

D1 ext

Muscle Fiber Types & Exercises to Increase Certain Muscle Fibers

Fiber Type	Common-Activity Muscles Most Active	Metabolic Capacity	Mitochondria	Exercises to ↑ Fiber Recruitment
Fast twitch, type IIb	Stop & go, all-out exercise requiring rapid, powerful movements	Anaerobic	Absent	Short duration, ↑ speed, heavy lifting
Fast oxidative glycolytic, IIa	Fast-contracting, longer duration	Combination of aerobic & anaerobic	Present	Combination of ↑ speed or wt & ↑ duration
Slow twitch, type I	Slow speed of contraction, continuous activity	Aerobic	Present	Long duration, ↓ wt, multiple repetitions in strength exercise

Guide to PT Practice Patterns for Musculoskeletal Conditions

Preferred Practice	Includes
Pattern 4A Primary prevention/risk reduction for skeletal demineralization	Prolonged non-weight-bearing; deconditioned, nutritional deficiency; menopause, hysterectomy, medications (e.g., steroids, thyroid medications); chronic cardiovascular & pulmonary dysfunction
Pattern 4B Impaired posture	Curvature of spine; disorders of back & neck; disk disorders; deformities of limbs; osteoporosis; muscle wasting; spasm; pregnancy-related problems; leg length discrepancy; joint stiffness
Pattern 4C Impaired muscle performance	Pelvic floor dysfunction, chronic neuromuscular dysfunction, loss of muscle strength & endurance, arthritis, transient paralysis
Pattern 4D Impaired joint mobility, motor function, muscle performance, & ROM associated w/*connective tissue dysfunction*	Joint subluxation or dislocation, ligament sprain, muscle sprain, prolonged immobilization, pain, swelling/effusion, arthritis, scleroderma, SLE
Pattern 4E Impaired joint mobility, motor function, muscle performance, & ROM associated w/*localized inflammation*	Ankylosing spondylitis, bursitis, capsulitis, epicondylitis, fascitis, gout, OA, synovitis, tendonitis, muscle strain/weakness
Pattern 4F Impaired joint mobility, motor function, muscle performance, ROM, & reflex integrity associated w/*spinal disorders*	Degenerative disk disease, spinal stenosis, spondylolisthesis, disk herniation, spinal surgery, ABN neural tension, altered sensation, muscle weakness, pain w/ forward bending

Continued

Guide to PT Practice Patterns for Musculoskeletal Conditions—cont'd

Preferred Practice	Includes
Pattern 4G Impaired joint mobility, muscle performance & ROM associated w/ *fracture*	Bone demineralization, fracture, hormonal changes, medications, prolonged non-weight bearing state, muscle weakness from immobilization, trauma
Pattern 4H Impaired joint mobility, motor function, muscle performance, & ROM associated w/*joint arthoplasty*	Arthoplastics, avascular necrosis, juvenile RA, neoplasms of the bone, OA, ankylosing spondylitis
Pattern 4I Impaired joint mobility, motor function, muscle performance, & ROM associated w/*bony or soft tissue surgery*	Fusions, ankylosis, bone graft & lengthening, caesarean section, connective tissue repair, fascial releases, internal débridement, intervertebral disk disorder, laminectomies, muscle or ligament repair, open reduction internal fixation, osteotomies
Pattern 4J Impaired joint mobility, motor function, muscle performance, ROM, gait, locomotion, & balance associated w/*amputation*	Amputation, frostbite, PVD, trauma

ICD-10 Codes for Skin & Subcutaneous Tissue

Diseases of the Skin & Subcutaneous Tissue

L00–L08 Infections of the skin and subcutaneous tissue
L10–L14 Bullous disorders
L20–L30 Dermatitis and eczema
L40–L45 Papulosquamous disorders
L49–L54 Urticaria and erythema
L55–L59 Radiation-related disorders of the skin and subcutaneous tissue
L60–L75 Disorders of skin appendages
L76   Intraoperative and postprocedural complications of skin and subcutaneous tissue
L80–L99 Other disorders of the skin and subcutaneous tissue

Assessment

Assessment of integumentary system includes:

- Activities, positioning, & postures that produce or relieve trauma to skin (observations, pressure-sensing maps, scales)
- Assistive, adaptive, orthotic, protective, supportive equipment that may produce or relieve trauma to skin
- Skin characteristics

  - Blistering
  - Nail growth
  - Continuity of skin color
  - Sensation
  - Dermatitis
  - Temperature
  - Hair growth
  - Texture
  - Mobility
  - Turgor
  - Pitting edema

- Burn description & quantification
- Wound characteristics

  - Bleeding
  - Shape
  - Contraction
  - Staging, progression, & etiology
  - Size
  - Depth
  - Location
  - Pulses/vascular tests

From World Health Organization. *International Statistical Classification of Diseases*, ed. 10. http://apps.who.int/classifications/icd10/browse/2010/en with permission.

- Drainage—serous, sanguinous, serosanguinous, or purulent
- Tunneling

- Exposed anatomical structures
- Undermining

- Wound scar tissue characteristics
  - Banding
  - Sensation
- Signs of infection
  - Cultures
  - Observations
  - Palpation

- Odor

- Periwound: girth, edema, etc.
- Pigment
- Pain
- Presence of granulation tissue or necrosis

- Pliability
- Texture

Classification of Burn Injury

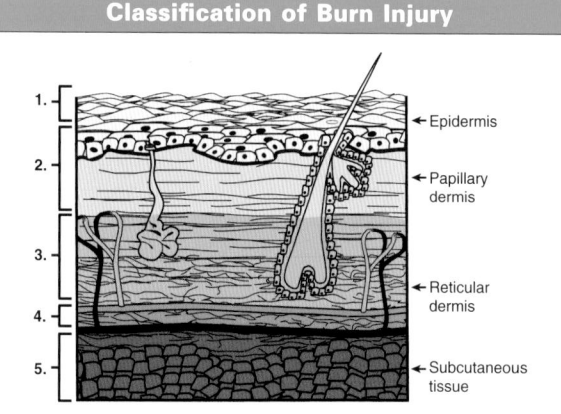

1. Superficial
2. Superficial partial thickness
3. Deep partial thickness
4. Full thickness
5. Subdermal

232

Classification of Burn Injury (cont'd)

Classification	Sensation	Blisters	Color	Appearance	Healing
Superficial	Pain/ tenderness delayed	Usually absent	Red	Dry, but edema may be present	Healing occurs w/o scarring
Superficial partial thickness	Severe pain	Intact blisters	Red	Bubbled w/blisters, edema	Minimal or no scarring
Deep partial thickness	Painful, but less severe than superficial	Broken	Mixed red or waxy white	Moderate edema/ WET from broken blisters	Healing occurs w/ hypertrophic scars & keloids
Full thickness	Anesthetic to pain & temp	None	White, brown, black, or red	Hard, parchment-like eschar formation or leathery, dry	Infection; grafts necessary/ skin regenerates only from edges of burn
Subdermal	Anesthetic	None	White, brown, black, or red	Necrotic tissue throughout	Extensive surgery necessary to remove necrotic tissue; may need to amputate

Types of Burn Injuries

Type	Cause	Wound Characteristics
Thermal burns	Skin exposed to flame	Wounds have irregular borders Depth of injury varies
	Sudden explosion or ignition of gases: flash burns	Exposed surfaces burned uniformly Usually result in partial-thickness burns
	Hot objects (metals): contact burns	Deep, sharply circumscribed wounds All skin elements & underlying structures destroyed
Scald burns	Contact w/hot liquids	Superficial wounds Hot liquid remains in contact w/skin for time (immersion/clothing holding liquid in contact), deep-partial or full-thickness injuries result
Chemical	From acids or strong alkalies	Tissue may be exposed for long periods unless washed immediately Result in partial- or full-thickness damage
Electrical	Electrical current	Cause well-circumscribed, deep injuries involving muscle, tendon, bone Neurovascular structures involved Injuries result in severe movement dysfunction & physical disability

Extent of Burned Area

Rule of Nines for Estimating Burn Area

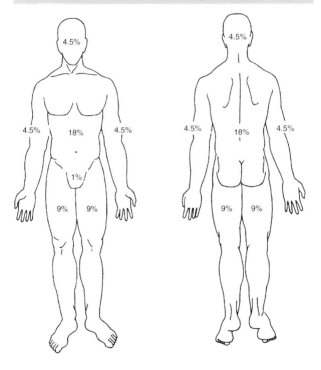

From Rothstein JM, Roy SH, Wolf SL. *The Rehabilitation Specialist's Handbook*, ed. 3. Philadelphia: FA Davis, 2005.

Secondary Complications of Burn Injury

2°	Description	Signs & Symptoms
Infection	Inflammation phase: ↑ risk of mortality: wound at risk due to ↑ edema, ↓ defense, & ↑ resistance to antibiotic Burns: systemic & topical antibiotics Wounds: topical antibiotics	Fever, lethargic, ↑ WBC Bacterial count >10^5 = wound infection; >10^7 associated w/↑ risk of mortality
Pulmonary	Suspect inhalation injury w/burn in a closed space (incidence >33%) or facial burns; ↑ risk of mortality Complications: CO poisoning, tracheal damage, upper airway obstruction, pulmonary edema, pneumonia Later complications: restrictive disease, inhalation injury, late sequelae (advanced restrictive disease) Perform xenon lung scan & serial PFT	Facial burns, singed nasal hairs, harsh cough, hoarseness, ABN breath sounds, respiration distress, sputum w/carbon, hypoxemia ↑ Risk of pneumonia
Metabolic	Rapid ↓ body wt, negative nitrogen balance, ↓ energy stores, change in glucose kinetics: result in hyperglycemia Treat w/nutrition, ↓ room temp	↑ Core temp, ↓ body wt, ↑ sweat & heat loss in room at NL temp; ↓ albumin, globulin, protein; ↑ free fatty acids, triglycerides
Cardiac Function/circulatory	Significant ↓ plasma & intravascular fluid volume; initial ↓ cardiac output (may ↓ 30% w/in first 30 min), alterations in platelet concentration & function, RBC dysfunction	↓ RBC, ↑ HR Deconditioning

Secondary Complications of Burn Injury—cont'd

2°	Description	Signs & Symptoms
Musculoskeletal	Significant damage to bone or peripheral circulation may result in amputation; significant ↓ wt results in loss of muscle mass & fiber atrophy	↓ Sarcomeres; ↓ ROM; muscle atrophy, osteoporosis, heterotopic ossification (pain, sudden loss of ROM w/in 3–12 wk after injury) Contractures
Neurological	Often seen in electrical injuries; involves spinal cord, brain, & peripheral nerves; often peripheral neuropathies; scar tissue formation may also cause nerve compression	Peripheral neuropathies, ↓ sensation, edema, ↓ strength
Pain	Pain limits spontaneous movement & exercise; when wound open: pain ↑; when wound closed: pain ↓; lubrication critical to avoid pain & skin crackling	Itching, ↑ sensitivity to heat, cold, touch

Burn Wound Healing

Area	Phase	Description
Dermal	Inflammatory	Begins time of injury; ends 3–5 d; leukocytes ↓ contamination; redness, edema, warmth, pain, ↓ ROM
	Proliferative	Surface: re-epithelial; deep: fibroblasts (cells synthesize scar tissue) migrate & proliferate; collagen deposited w/random alignment; stresses (stretching): fibers align along path of stress Granulation tissue formed: blood vessels, macrophages, fibroblasts Wound contraction occurs; skin grafts may ↓ contracture
	Maturation	Remodeling of scar: 2 y/↓ in fibroblasts, vasculitis ↓, collagen remodels, & ↑ strength; hypertrophic scar: red, raised, firm; rate of collagen production > rate of collagen breakdown Keloid: large, firm scar/overflows wound boundaries
Epidermal		Wound surface: cells migrate & cover wound; damage to sebaceous glands may cause dryness & itching during healing; external lubrication needed

Classification of Ulcers

Etiology	Location	Defining Characteristics
Vascular ulcers: arterial	Distal lower extremities: toes, feet, shin	Pain: severe unless neuropathy masking pain Gangrene: may be present Signs: ↓ pulses, trophic changes, cyanosis when dependent
Vascular ulcers: venous insufficiency Tracing to assess wound size	Distal lower extremities: inner or outer ankle	Pain: not severe Surrounding skin: pigmented, fibrotic Gangrene: absent Signs: edema, stasis dermatitis
Trophic ulcers (decubitus or pressure sores): usually due to impaired sensation	Over bony prominences: areas w/diminished sensation; usually secondary to immobilization	Pain: absent Surrounding skin: callous Signs: ↓ sensation, ↓ ankle jerks
Diabetic foot ulcers	Distal position: around toes, deep into foot	Highly aggressive & may lead to serious complications, amputations ↑ risk of infection

Clinical Indicators for Differentiating Arterial vs. Venous Wounds

Arterial	Venous
Intermittent claudication	Localized limb pain: ↓ w/elevation, ↑ w/standing
Extreme pain	Pain w/deep pressure or palpation
↓ or absent pedal pulses	Pedal pulses present
↓ temp of distal limb	↑ temp around wound
Well-defined wound edges	Nondistinct, irregular edges
Deep wound bed	Shallow wound bed
Cyanosis	Edema around the wound Substantial drainage

Stages & Etiology of Pressure Wounds

Stage	Description	Etiology: Out→Inside	Etiology: Inside→Out
I	Redness (discoloration in pigment skin) w/o breakdown & will not blanch; warm, edema, induration, or hardness	Pressure to skin distorts superficial blood vessels: ischemia & leakage	Pressure on deep muscle decreases blood flow to skin
II	Partial-thickness skin loss (epidermis, dermis, or both), abrasion, blister/ shallow crater	Prolonged superficial pressure leads to more necrosis	Pressure on perforators is extensive, leading to ↓ blood flow to skin

Stages & Etiology of Pressure Wounds—cont'd

Stage	Description	Etiology: Out→Inside	Etiology: Inside→Out
III	Full-thickness skin loss, damage or necrosis to subcutaneous tissue, may extend to underlying fascia; presents as deep crater w/ or w/o undermining tissue	Persistent external pressure	Distortion of deep blood vessels by pressure of bone or muscle impairs blood flow
IV	Full-thickness skin loss w/↑ tissue necrosis/damage to muscle w/ exposed bone or supporting tissues; undermining	Extremely high pressure & prolonged: affects deep blood vessels	Prolonged pressure on blood vessels is severe; muscle necrosis

(AHCPR, 2012)

Wound Characteristics From Wound Bed Assessment

Characteristics	Indications	Diagnostic Technique	Concerns/Additional Comments
Color	Look for signs of clinical infection Evaluate progress of therapeutic regimen	Photos & color coding: look at black, yellow, red areas; analyze color by computer software; w/o software, use pictures	Maintain standard protocol: Same camera Same lighting Same distance from wound Same flash on camera

Continued

Characteristics	Indications	Diagnostic Technique	Concerns/ Additional Comments
Odor	Assessment of bacteria	Electronic noses Clinical: description of odor	Electronic nose $$$; not found in clinic Odor doesn't identify specific bacteria involved
Temp	↑ Temp associated w/ infection ↓ Temp slows healing: ↓ O_2 release Chronic leg wounds: 24°C–26°C	Infrared thermography Glass mercury thermometers or electronic display devices using thermistors	$$$/not widely available in clinic Thermometers: more easily understood & more widely used
pH	Intact skin: 4.8–6.0, interstitial fluid = neutral pH monitors healing: acidification from chemicals ↑ healing	Flat glass electrode	Wound pH measurement used to predict skin graft survival, wound healing under synthetic dressings, etc.
Area & volume	Defines progress of healing	3D mapping from scanned images; clinical use of photos/tracings of wound & depth measures	Recorded at baseline & weekly intervals

Risk Factors for Pressure Ulcers

Risk Factor	Preventive Actions
Bed/chair confinement	Inspect skin 1 ×/day; bathe daily, prevent dry skin Avoid use of doughnut-shaped cushions; participate in rehabilitation program ↓ friction on skin by lifting (do not drag) & cornstarch on skin

	Bed Confinement	Chair Confinement
	Change position q 2 h	Change position q 1 h
	Use foam, air, gel, H_2O mattress	Use foam, gel, or air cushion

Risk Factor	Preventive Actions
Inability to move	Reposition q h. Change position q 15 min if cannot shift wt in chair Use pillows/wedges to keep knees & ankles from touching Place pillow under midcalf in bed to keep heels from touching
Loss of bowel or bladder control	Clean skin whenever soiled/assess & treat urine leaks If constant moisture: use absorbent pads w/quick-drying surface Protect skin w/cream or ointment
Poor nutrition	Eat balanced diet/consider nutritional supplement
↓ mental awareness	Choose preventive actions that apply If confined to bed or chair, change position as noted above

Identifying Skin Cancers

Cancers	Etiology	Warning Signs
Malignant melanoma: one of most virulent cancers Courtesy of Dr. Benjamin Barankin.	Excessive exposure to sun Heredity Atypical moles	Change in surface of a mole: Scaliness/oozing/bleeding Spread of pigment from border → surrounding skin Change in sensation (itchiness, tenderness, pain)
Basal cell carcinoma Courtesy of Dr. Benjamin Barankin.	Most common cancer in whites Risk factors: light hair, eyes, complexions; tan poorly	Fleshy bump or nodule on head, neck, or hands: rarely metastasizes but can extend below skin
Squamous cell carcinoma	Second most common skin cancer found in whites Develops into large masses: can metastasize	Appears as nodules or red, scaly patches; found on rim of ear, face, lips, & mouth

Other Skin Problems

Psoriasis.

Etiology: Genetic/noncontagious; appears as a result of a "trigger": Emotional stress, injury to skin, drug reaction, some infections

Warning Signs: Generalized fatigue, tenderness/swelling or pain over tendons, morning stiffness, redness & rash, swollen fingers/toes

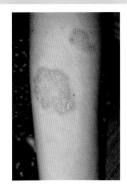

Courtesy of Dr. Benjamin Barankin.

Cellulitis.

Etiology: Acute inflammation with infection that spreads rapidly due to *Streptococcus pyogenes* or *Staphylococcus aureus,* or *Haemophilus influenzae* in children

Warning Signs: Red, tender or painful, edematous, warm, ↑ WBCs; at risk if low resistance

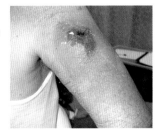

From *Derm Notes*: B Barankin and A Freiman FA Davis; Philadelphia; 2006 p. 74.

Shingles (herpes zoster).

Etiology: Dormant varicella zoster virus (chicken pox) reactivates, often due to immunosuppression or stress.

Warning Signs: Pain/tenderness along dermatome (unilateral) followed by rash, papules, & crusting over 2–4 wk period

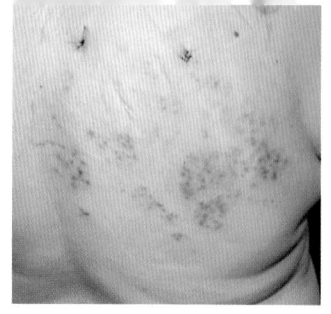

From *Derm Notes*: B Barankin and A Freiman FA Davis; Philadelphia; 2006 p. 100.

Methicillin-resistant *Staphylococcus aureus* (MRSA)

Etiology: Misuse or overuse of antibiotics causes resistant infections, and poor hand washing causes fast spread of infection

Warning Signs: Fever, chills, sweating, malaise, confusion

Other Risk Factors in Wound Care

- Circulation: poor circulation increases risk
- Chemotherapy: overall cell destruction
- Steroid therapy: ↓ inflammatory response
- Presence of systemic infection
- Diabetes: ↓ circulation & sensation
- Repeated trauma: ↑ friction injury
- ↓ age: ↓ epithelial turnover & elasticity
- ↓ albumin &/or ↓ prealbumin: malnutrition

Interventions

Topical Meds Frequently Used in Burn Treatment

Med	Description	Application
Polysporin (bacitracin)	Clear ointment; used for gram-positive infections	Small amount applied directly to wound: keep uncovered
Accuzyme (collagenase)	Enzymatic débriding (necrotic tissue selectively); no antibacterial effects	Apply to eschar, cover w/ moist dressing w/ or w/o antibacterial agent
Furacin (nitrofurazone)	Antibacterial cream for less severe burns; ↓ bacterial growth	Applied directly on wound or gauze dressing
Gentamicin	Antibiotic for gram-negative, staph & strep bacteria	Applied w/sterile glove; covered w/gauze
Silver sulfadiazine	Most commonly used antibacterial agent; used especially for *Pseudomonas*	White cream applied w/ sterile glove 2–4 mm thick to wound or into mesh gauze; may be left open
Sulfamylon (mafenide acetate)	Topical antibacterial; used for gram-negative or -positive; diffuses through eschar	White cream applied directly to wound (1–2 mm thick) 2 ×/d; left open or w/thin layer of gauze
Silver nitrate	Antiseptic germicide & cleanser, penetrates only 1–2 mm eschar; for surface bacteria; stains black	Used every 2 h in dressings or soaks; also available in small sticks
Scar treatment medications: 1. Cica-Care Gel Sheets 2. Mederma	1. Silicone gel that flattens & softens scars 2. Topical gel to reduce visibility of scars	1. One sheet lasts 28 d 2. Rub 3–4 ×/d for 3–6 mo

Commonly Used Dressings for Burn Wounds, Skin Grafts, & Donor Sites

Dressings	Category	Examples	Indications
Nonbiologic	Petrolatum	Xeroform, Xeroflo, Adaptic, Aquaphor gauze	Partial-thickness burns, skin grafts, donor sites
	Silver	Acticoat, Acticoat-7 Aquacel-Ag, Silvasorb	Partial-thickness burns, skin grafts, donor sites
	Polyurethane	OpSite, Tegaderm	Partial-thickness burns, donor sites
	Foam	Lyofoam	Partial-thickness burns
	Silicone	Mepitel	Partial-thickness burns, skin grafts, donor sites
	Negative pressure therapy	Wound VAC system	Skin grafts
Biosynthetic & biologic	Oat	Glucan II	Partial-thickness burns, skin grafts, donor sites
	Collagen & fibroblasts	Transcyte, Apligraf	Partial-thickness burns
	Collagen, fibroblasts, & keratinocytes	OrCel	Partial-thickness burns
	Allograft (cadaver)	Fresh or cryopreserved	Partial-thickness burns
	Xenograft	Porcine skin, porcine intestinal submucosa (oasis)	Partial-thickness burns

Adapted from Pham TN, Gibran NS. Thermal and Electrical Injuries, *Surg Clin N Am* 2007;87(1):185–206 and from Paz, West, Jaime C., Michele C. *Acute Care Handbook for Physical Therapists*, ed 3. W.B. Philadelphia: Saunders Company, 2009. 7.5.1.

Wound Dressings/Treatments*

Dressings	Brand Name	Clinical Tips
Thin films (polyurethane films)	Opsite Tegaderm Polyskin Bioclusive	For stage I, II w/minimal drainage, NO infection Nonabsorbent, permeable to gas, contraindicated on fragile skin, works well w/moist dressings, works over joints
Hydrocolloid	Comfeel Plus Ulcer Dressing Comfeel Plus Transparent Dressing Granuflex Bordered DuoDerm Extra Thin Tegasorb	For stage I, II, III w/minimal to moderate drainage & NO infection Aggressive adhesion, not effective in dry wounds Difficult to visualize surrounding skin Moderately absorbent Not indicated in stage IV
Alginate/CMC fibrous dressing	SeaSorb Soft dressing Aquacel dressing Sorbsan dressing	For stage II, III, IV w/moderate to excessive wound drainage Absorbs exudates, maintains wound moisture, semipermeable, requires 2nd dressing & careful removal

Continued

Dressings	Brand Name	Clinical Tips
Hydrogels	Purilon gel IntraSite gel Duoderm Hydroactive gel Solosite Vigilon	For stage II, III, IV, & nonstageable w/minimal drainage, NO infection Assists in débridement by hydration; nonadherent; difficult to keep in place ↓ pain, closes naturally; requires a secondary dressing, semipermeable
Foam dressings	Blatain Non-adhesive Blatain Adhesive Allevyn Non-adhesive Allevyn Adhesive Mepilex Mepilex border	For stage III, IV w/excessive drainage & NO infection Nonadherent, absorbs large amount exudates; semipermeable
Absorptive dressings (granular exudate absorbers)	Bard Absorption Dressing Hydragan Debrisan	For stage III, IV w/wound drainage, NO infection Good filler for deep wounds, keeps moist, used to débride w/autolysis Difficult to keep in place, requires 2nd dressing, semipermeable

*Wound dressings are constantly revised & newer ones may be available.

Wound Débridement

Type of Débridement			Benefits/Precautions
Selective			
Sharp	Use of scalpels, scissors, forceps, hydrosurgery, or lasers	Expedient in removal of large, thick, leathery eschar	↑ degree of wound healing 1. Can be painful 2. Can cause excessive bleeding
Autolytic	Apply moisture-retentive topical dressing: films, hydrocolloids, hydrogels, & calcium alginates	Takes time for this type, but natural & painless	Contraindicated as primary débridement in immunosuppressed patient/clients
Enzymatic	Topical application of enzymes that lyse collagen, fibrin, & elastin: proteolytics, fibrinolytics, & collagenases	Used for stage II & IV but discontinued when wound clean	Metals like zinc oxide & silver in cleansing agents can interfere & inactivate enzymes
Nonselective			
Mechanical	Dry gauze bandages, whirlpool, pulsed lavage, or irrigation	Wet to dry dressings débride by taking necrotic tissue embedded Pulsed lavage best for incontinent patient/clients	Don't use on clean, granulating wounds Caution with temp of whirlpool water, time in water, position of extremity so as not to increase swelling

Skin Grafts & Flaps Used in Burn Treatment

Skin Graft/Flap	Description
Advancement flap	Local flap; skin next to wound moved to cover defect w/detachment from original site
Allograft (homograft, cadaver)	Taken from donor but not genetically identical to recipient
Autograft	Taken from recipient's body
Delayed graft	Partially elevated & replaced: moved to another site
Free flap	Skin tissue moved to a distant site where vascular reconnection is made
Full-thickness graft	Contains all skin layers but no subcutaneous fat
Heterograft	Taken from member of another species
Isologous	From donor genetically identical to recipient
Local flap	Relocation of skin to adjacent site w/part of flap remaining attached to own blood supply
Mesh graft	Donor's skin cut to form mesh: expanded to cover a larger area
Myocutaneous flap	Flap w/muscle, subcutaneous fat, skin, & patent blood supply
Pedical flap	Flap w/one end attached: allows blood supply to reconnect new end
Rotational flap/Z-plasty	Local flap: section incised on three sides & pivoted: covers area next to it
Sheet graft	Donor skin applied w/o alteration to recipient's damaged area
Split-thickness graft	Graft w/only superficial dermal layers

Physical Therapy Intervention per Healing Phase

Inflammation	Proliferation & Migration Phase	Remodeling & Maturation Phase
0 to 5 d	5 to 21 d/up to 6 wk	6 wk to 6 mo/up to 1 y
Protection Phase	**Controlled Motion Phase**	**Return to Function Phase**
Control effects of inflammation (pain, edema, spasm)	Promote healing & monitor response of healing tissue	↑ strength & alignment of scar
Selective rest/immobilization	Nondestructive active, resistive, open/closed chain stabilization, muscle endurance	Progressive stretching, strengthening, endurance training, functional exercises, and specificity drills
Promote early healing & prevent negative effect of rest	Progress PROM to AAROM to AROM	↑ tissue mobility
Passive movement, massage, muscle setting (isometrics)	Multiple-angle isometric exercise	Stretching: joint mobilization, cross fiber massage, neuromuscular inhibition, passive stretch, massage
AAROM, resistive, modified aerobic in other areas	If ROM improved, progress isotonic exercise	Progress exercise: resistance; simple to complex, increase time
Proper dosage of rest & movement	Resume low-intensity functional activities	Progress aerobic exercise
Contraindicated—stretching & resistance exercise of inflamed tissue	Inflammation should be ↓; if patient/client has pain lasting >2 hr, it is too much	Progressive functional activities w/less protective support
	Too much—resting pain, fatigue, increased weakness, spasm	Should be no signs of inflammation
		↑ intensity of exercise if patient/client returning to high-demand activities; plyometrics, agility training, skill

Hayes, D. From course materials for Medical Physiology, North Georgia College and State University.

Positioning for Common Deformities

Common Joint	Deformity	Motions to Be Stressed	Approaches to Positioning
Neck: anterior	Flexion	Hyperextension	Position neck in extension or use rigid cervical orthosis
Shoulder/axilla	Adduction/internal rotation	Abduction, flexion, external rotation	Position w/shoulder flexed & abducted
Elbow	Flexion/pronation	Extension/supination	Splint in extension
Hand	Claw hand (intrinsic minus)	Wrist extension, MCP flexion, proximal & distal ICP extension, thumb in palmar abduction	Wrap fingers individually, elevate for edema; use intrinsic positive, wrist in extension, MCP flexion, proximal & distal ICP in extension, thumb in palmar abduction w/web space
Hip/groin	Flexion/adduction	All motions, especially hip extension, abduction	Hip neutral, extension w/slight abduction
Knee	Flexion	Extension	Posterior knee splint
Ankle	Plantar flexion	All motions	Plastic ankle-foot orthosis, ankle positioned in 0° dorsiflexion

Positioning for Common Deformities *(continued)*

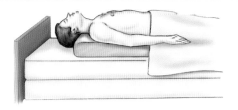

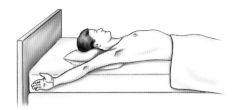

Electrotherapy Treatments for Burns/Wounds

Modality	Indication
Infrared	Fungal infections, psoriatic lesions
Hydrotherapy	Cleanse & enhance wound healing
Electric stimulation	To enhance wound healing

Adjunctive Interventions in Wound Healing

Intervention	Description	Contraindications
Normothermia	Delivery of warm, moist heat from infrared heating element inserted into dressing; treatment: three 1-h treatments/d	Cannot be used on 3rd-degree burns
Intervention: UV radiation therapy	UV lamp plus commercial product: derma wand or Handisol; use UV depending on desired treatment effect	TB, systemic diseases (renal, liver, cardiac, or lupus), cancer in wound, fever, acute psoriasis, herpes simplex, or eczema
Intervention: negative pressure therapy	Apply controlled level of subatmospheric pressure (5–125 mm Hg < ambient pressure) to interior of wound; open cell polyurethane foam dressing, apply via pump in continuous vacuum	None

Adjunctive Interventions in Wound Healing—cont'd

Intervention	Description	Contraindications
Intervention: hyperbaric O_2 therapy	Patient/client breathes OR tissue is surrounded by 100% O_2 at pressures > NL atmospheric pressure (O_2 delivery 2–3 × > atmospheric pressure); indications: gas gangrene, problem wounds, necrotizing soft tissue infection, osteomyelitis, thermal burns, crush injuries	Seizure disorders, malignant tumor Toxic effects if used improperly: S & S of O_2 toxicity: dry cough, nausea/vomiting, pulmonary fibrosis, visual changes, seizures
Intervention: platelet-derived growth factor	Topically applied bioengineered growth factor to accelerate healing; particularly for diabetic foot ulcer	Limited evidence of efficacy on wounds except diabetic foot
Intervention: stem cell therapy	Pluripotential stem cells differentiate into fibroblasts, endothelial cells, & keratinocytes	Found in bone marrow: currently controversy exists w/use of stem cells

Scar Management Techniques

- Healing of deeper burns and skin-grafted burns is accompanied by some scarring.
- Hypertrophic scarring can be decreased by the use of pressure garments, silicone gel sheets, ROM, and massage.

Guccione, 2012.

Scar Management

Tools	Description	Limitations/Benefits
Scar massage	Performed several times/day Utilize bland moisturizers, which limit drying; massage in firm, slow manner	Benefit: can be performed by multiple people Limitation: large areas
Ultrasonic or microwave heating	Softens scar & loosens stiff joints. ↓ tensile strength of scar, reduces collagen content	Benefit seen in half of all patient/clients
Compression garments	Improves control of broad areas of scarring Worn 23 h/d for 12–18 mo after injury	Must refit & replace if poor fit or growing child
Topical silicone	Applied as a sheet Effective for small areas Keep in place 24 h/d	Rash possible. Need to cut time sheet is on Firm pressure not req
Steroid injections	For localized symptomatic areas of scars, for cosmetic areas, or when pruritis develops	Dose needs to be limited to prevent systemic effects Painful
Surgical excision or incision & autografting or Z-plasty	For burn deformities that scar mgmt tools have not helped	Few surgeries necessary 1st year after injury High priority for contractures around mouth or neck that interfere w/airway
Laser surgery	Laser beam causes a thermal tissue reaction Flashlamp-pumped pulse dye laser results in less pruritic, more pliable, less erythematous scar	CO_2 & argon lasers are ineffective
Cryotherapy	Causes microcirculatory disturbances that lead to tissue damage	Keloids do not respond as well

Practice Patterns of Integumentary Disorders

No.	Practice Patterns	Includes Individuals With
7A	Primary prevention/risk reduction for integumentary disorders	Amputation, CHF, diabetes, malnutrition, neuromuscular dysfunction, obesity, peripheral nerve involve, polyneuropathy, prior scar, SCI, surgery, vascular disease
7B	Impaired integumentary integrity associated w/superficial skin involvement	Amputation, burns (superficial & 1st degree), cellulitis, contusion, dermopathy, dermatitis, malnutrition, neuropathic ulcers (grade 0), pressure ulcers (grade 2), vascular disease (arterial, diabetic, venous)
7C	Impaired integumentary integrity associated w/partial-thickness skin involvement & scar formation	Amputation, burns, derm disorders, epidermolysis bullosa, hematoma, immature scar, malnutrition, neoplasm, neuropathic ulcer, pressure ulcer, prior scar, s/p post-SCI, surgical wounds, toxic epidermal necrolysis, traumatic injury, vascular ulcers
7D	Impaired integumentary integrity associated w/full-thickness skin involvement & scar formation	Amputation, burns, frostbite, hematoma, scar (immature, hypertrophic, or keloid), lymphostatic ulcer, malnutrition, neoplasm, neuropathic ulcers, pressure ulcers, surgical wounds, toxic epidermal necrolysis, vascular ulcers
7E	Impaired integumentary integrity associated w/skin involvement extending into fascia, muscle, or bone & scar formation	Abscess, burns, chronic surgical wounds, electric burns, frostbite, hematoma, Kaposi sarcoma, lymphostatic ulcer, necrotizing fasciitis, neoplasm, neuropathic ulcers (grades 3, 4, 5), pressure ulcers (stage 4), recent amputation, subcutaneous arterial ulcer, surgical wounds, vascular ulcers

APTA: Guide to Physical Therapist Practice ed. 2. *Physical Therapy* 2001;81:9–744.

Daily Assessments

Assessment (check daily)	YES/NO	Changes Noted
New symptoms?		
Worsening symptoms? Describe		
Medication changes?		
Vital signs: significant differences from previous visit?		
Lab values: any new changes?		
Daily weight change? Check patient/client's log (especially for heart failure or COPD patient/clients)		
Skin changes?		
Activity changes?		
Changes in sleep patterns or amt of sleep?		
Recent visit to MD or ER and any changes since visit?		
Changes in equipment needs?		
Changes in caregiver needs?		
Obstacles to performing activities?		
Dietary needs/recommendations?		

Assessment

Measures More Frequently Used in the Home Setting

Outcome Measure	Target of Measurement
Borg Rating of Perceived Exertion	Perceived effort w/activity (6–20 scale or 0–10 scale)
Chair Rise test	Functional lower extremity strength assessment
Falls assessment (see Neuro Tab)	Determine risk for falls
Gait Speed Test (see Cardio Tab)	Compare gait speed to functional indicators such as falls risk, risk for rehospitalization, etc
Modified Romberg (see Neuro Tab)	Balance screen
Short Physical Performance Battery	Balance, lower extremity functional strength, & gait speed measurements to screen for functional assessment
Timed Walk Tests (3-, 6-, 12-min)	Functional performance during ambulation: originally tested in chronic lung disease patient/clients
Timed Stands Test	Lower extremity strength in patient/clients w/arthritis
Timed "Up and Go" Test	Mobility of frail elderly: timed rise from chair, walk for 3 m, return to sit
Visual Analogue Scale for Dyspnea	Patient/client's perceptions of dyspnea; used w/activities

Assistive/Adaptive Equipment Assessment in Home

Identified Dysfunction	Equipment to Consider	Assessment of Equipment
Unable to ambulate for distances	Wheelchair	Assess height, weight, & buttocks width to determine size of chair Assess need for removable arms/legs & reclining back or legs Assess comfort in w/c (see Assessment Tab for w/c measurement)
	Wheeled walker, regular walker, cane Mobility scooter	Assess individual's height & height at hand grip w/30° bend in elbow Scooter: assess body height, leg height, hip to knee length, arm reach to handlebars
Difficulty getting up from bed to stand, needs multiple pillows to sleep	Bed risers Bed rails, trapeze, poles, or grab bars Electric bed to raise head or feet up or raise or lower from floor	Assess ability to get up from elevated height—may only need risers Assess ability to hold on to bed assists
Difficulty standing up from low chairs	Higher height chair or a motorized lift chair Poles to use for standing from sit	Evaluate heights from which individual can rise to standing & heights that are difficult Determine amount of assist needed to stand
Difficulty rising up from toilet	Elevated toilet seat Hand rails around toilet to help with push	Assess heights from which individual rise to standing & heights that are difficult Assess amount of assist needed

Assistive/Adaptive Equipment Assessment in Home—cont'd

Identified Dysfunction	Equipment to Consider	Assessment of Equipment
Skin breakdown on buttocks	Specialized cushions, including ROHO or gel	Evaluate the length of time patient/client is sitting in chair to determine special cushion and need for skin-protective garments
Other skin breakdown	Bolsters & pillows	Evaluate skin healing
Difficulty standing in shower for lengths of time; unable to get in tub	Shower bench Wheeled shower chair	Evaluate bathroom and need for grab bars, whether tub or standing shower w/curb

Interventions

- Progressive aerobic activity
- Functional strengthening
- Transfer training for chairs, bed, bathroom, car
- Breathing exercises
- Stretching/flexibility activities
- Discussion of dietary needs including recommendations
- Education on:
  - Skin inspection
  - Daily weights
  - Symptom monitoring
  - Changes in temp, breathing, sleeping, cough, and sputum
  - Energy conservation
  - Use of adaptive or assistive equipment
  - Signs of exercise/activity intolerance
  - Prevention of other impairment

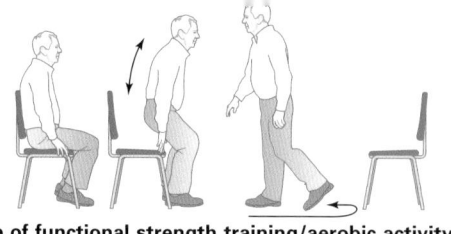

Example of functional strength training/aerobic activity combined.

Individual should work on rising from chair, taking short walk, and then turning around and sitting back down. Perform activities multiple times. When distance walked between chairs gets easier, increase distance between chairs.

Heart Failure Home Program

Patient/clients with heart failure require specific daily assessments.

Assessment	Indicators
Daily weight	↑ 2–3 lb overnight: auscultation of lungs, contact MD/NP/RN
Perceived exertion with all activities	↑ Perceived exertion with activities: auscultation of lungs, contact MD/NP/RN
Sx at rest and/or increased with activity	↑ in Sx: auscultation of lungs, contact MD/NP/RN
Sleep positions	↑ # pillows need to sleep or recliner needed: auscultation of lungs, contact MD/NP/RN
Peripheral edema: hands, feet, abdomen, JVD	↑ in edema: contact MD/NP/RN
Gait speed	↓ in gait speed of 0.1 m/sec is a significant change indicating ↓ in function: contact MD/NP/RN
Exercise tolerance	↓ in exercise tolerance: auscultation of lungs, check meds, contact MD/NP/RN

COPD Program

Assessment	Indicators
Sputum color change or amount	Sputum color change to yellow/green: auscultation of lungs, check temp, contact MD/NP/RN
SOB/dyspnea at rest or with activities	Dyspnea scale reporting different w/rest or activity, contact MD/NP/RN
Sleep position	↑ # of pillows needed for sleep or recliner needed: auscultation of lung sounds, contact MD/NP/RN
SpO$_2$ decreases at rest or w/activity that is different from previous visits	SpO$_2$ is lower than previously at rest &/or w/activity, contact MD/NP/RN
Exercise tolerance	↓ with increased Sx: determine any difference from previous visit, possibly contact MD/NP/RN

Diabetes

Assessment	Indicators of Concern
Daily blood sugars (fasting or not)	<100 at rest or w/activity >250 at rest or w/activity > normal
Sx at rest or w/activity; especially SOB or fatigue Other Sx to monitor • Chest tightness • Arm or jaw discomfort • Dizziness • Indigestion • Posterior shoulder blade discomfort	When Sx wake patient/client in middle of night, or ↑ w/activity, or do not diminish w/rest, contact MD/NP/RN
Exercise tolerance	When ↓ compared to previously, re-evaluate
Skin	*Any* open wound, contact RN/NP/MD
Medication changes	Patient/client demonstrates ↑ Sx and Sx are affecting function, contact MD/NP/RN

ICD 10 Codes Commonly Used With Women's Health

N00–N99 Diseases of the Genitourinary System
N00–N08 Glomerular diseases
N10–N16 Renal tubulo-interstitial diseases
N17–N19 Renal failure
N20–N23 Urolithiasis
N25–N29 Other disorders of kidney and ureter
N30–N39 Other diseases of urinary system
N60–N64 Disorders of breast
N70–N77 Inflammatory diseases of female pelvic organs
N80–N98 Noninflammatory disorders of female genital tract
N99 Other disorders of genitourinary tract

O00–O99 Pregnancy, Childbirth, and the Puerperium
O00–O08 Pregnancy with abortive outcome
O10–O16 Edema, proteinuria, and hypertensive disorders in pregnancy, childbirth, and the puerperium
O20–O29 Other maternal disorders predominantly related to pregnancy
O30–O48 Maternal care related to the fetus and amniotic cavity and possible delivery problems
O60–O75 Complications of labor and delivery
O80–O84 Delivery
O85–O92 Complications predominantly related to the puerperium
O94–O99 Other obstetric conditions, not elsewhere classified

Quick Screen for Women's Health Dysfunction

See the sections that follow for the entire screen. The following should be performed on all women:

- Breast health screening
- Risk factors for heart disease
- Risk factors for osteoporosis
- Risk factors for pelvic floor dysfunction
- Risk factors for pregnancy-induced pathology
- High-risk conditions in pregnancy

From World Health Organization. *International Statistical Classification of Diseases*, ed. 10. http://apps.who.int/classifications/icd10/browse/2010/en with permission.

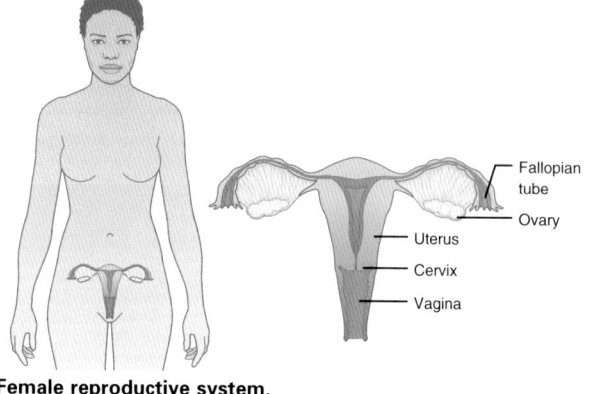

Female reproductive system.

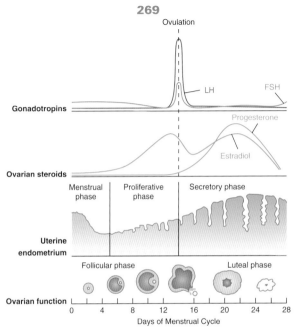

The hormonal levels during a normal menstrual cycle.

Fetal Growth & Changes During Pregnancy

Trimester/ Weeks	Fetus	Mother
FIRST 0 through 12	Implantation of fertilized egg @ 7–10 d after fertilization Fetus growth approx 6–7 cm & 2 oz Fetus has heartbeat, can kick, turn head, swallow	↑ Fatigue Urination frequency Possible nausea & vomiting ↑ in breast size Wt gain of ≤3 lb ↑ in emotionality
SECOND 13 through 26	Fetus growth approx 19–23 cm; wt 1–2 lb Fetus has eyebrows, eyelashes, fingernails	Visible growth of abdomen (growth of baby) Movement felt by 20 wk
THIRD 27 through 40	By birth, baby 33–39 cm; wt 5–10 lb	Uterus large Contractions occur often but felt occasionally Mother c/o frequent urination, back pain, leg edema, fatigue, round ligament pain, SOB, constipation
Labor	Stage 1: cervical dilation & effacement Stage 2: position changes, pushing, & expulsion Stage 3: expulsion of placenta, uterus contracts & ↓ in size for 3–6 wk post delivery	

Anatomical/Physiological Changes of Pregnancy

Systems/Body	Changes	Risk
Weight	↑ in wt 25–27 lb	May gain excess wt ↑ Risk obesity
Uterus & connective tissue	Uterus ↑ 5–6 × in size, 20 × in Vwt Ureters enter bladder perpendicular due to ↑ uterine size	↑ Risk of urinary tract infections ↑ Risk of ligament laxity & ↑ risk of injury
Pulmonary	↑ in upper respiratory hypersecretion due to hormones AP & transverse chest diameters ↑ Diaphragm elevated ↑ Depth of respiration (↑ TV, minute vent) ↑ O_2 consumption (15%–20%) Dyspnea w/exercise by 20 wk	↑ Work of breathing w/↑ RR Late in pregnancy: ↑ SOB w/lying flat
Cardiovascular, including blood volume & pressure	Volume ↑ 35%–50%; returns to normal 6–8 wk after birth (plasma volume) Venous pressure ↑ in LEs; ↑ pressure in inferior vena cava BP ↓ ↑ Heart rhythm disturbances ↑ HR (10–20 beats/min) CO ↑ 30%–60%	↑ Risk of venous distensibility; varicose veins & DVT ↑ Risk of decrease in CO when supine: symptomatic supine hypotension syndrome ↑ Risk of ventricular hypertrophy

Continued

Systems/Body	Changes	Risk
Muscles	Abdominal: muscle stretching ↓ ability to generate strong contraction Pelvic floor: drops 1 in Joint hypermobility ↑ Stretch on connective tissue & ligaments ↓ in ligamentous tensile strength	↑ Risk of injury
Thermoregulatory system	↑ BMR ↑ Heat production increase	Need to ↑ calorie intake by 300/d
Posture/Balance	Center of gravity shifts up & forward ↑ in lumbar & cervical lordoses Shoulder girdle & upper back more rounded, UE internally rotated ↑ Base of support of LE	↑ Risk of back/neck pain ↑ Risk of pectoralis tightness & scapular weakness ↑ Problems w/fine balance & rapid direction change activities

High-Risk Pregnancy Conditions Requiring Specialized Care

- Preterm rupture of membranes
- Premature onset of labor (<37 weeks)
- Incompetent cervix
- Placenta previa (placenta attaches too low on cervix)
- Pregnancy hypertension or pre-eclampsia
- Multiple gestation
- Diabetes

Pregnancy-Induced Pathologies

Pathology	Problems	Examination	Intervention
Diastasis recti (may also be due to postpartum)	Low back pain Unable to perform supine to sit Less protection for fetus Potential abdominal visceral herniation	Test frequently & after 3rd day postpartum Test in hook-lying position Patient/client raises head & shoulders off floor, reaches hands to knees until scapula spine leaves floor Patient/client places fingers horizontally across midline at umbilicus to check for separation & sinking of fingers; test above, at, & below umbilicus Record number of fingers placed between muscle bellies	Patient/client crosses arms at or below umbilicus & pulls rectus toward midline while raising head Goal is to ↓ separation to 2 cm Once separation is ↓, strengthen obliques & advanced abdominal activities

Continued

Pathology	Problems	Examination	Intervention
Postural back pain	Low back pain ↑ w/muscle fatigue as day progresses	Take a history of pain Assess all motion	Stabilization or therapeutic exercises & proper body mechanics Postural instructions; superficial modalities can be used
Sacroiliac/ pelvic girdle pain	Posterior pelvic pain Stabbing, deep buttock pain distal & lateral to L5/ S1 Pain w/ prolonged sitting, standing, walking, climbing stairs, turn in bed, unilateral stand Worsens w/ activity	Assess history & symptoms Palpation of areas of pain	Activity modification Exercise modifications (no excessive hip abduction or hyperextension) Stabilization exercises External stabilization w/ belt or corset

Pregnancy-Induced Pathologies—cont'd

Pathology	Problems	Examination	Intervention
Varicose veins	Symptoms of heaviness or aching in LEs in dependent leg positions Risk of DVT	Assess symptoms, leg edema possibly Doppler or ultrasound for DVT	Reduce dependent position/ prolonged standing Elastic support stockings to provide external pressure gradient against distended veins
Joint laxity	All joints are at ↑ risk of injury until months after delivery	Assess symptoms & ligament integrity	Instruct in safe exercises to ↓ stress on joints Non-weight-bearing or low-impact exercise
Nerve compression syndromes	Thoracic outlet syndrome (TOS) Carpal tunnel syndrome (CTS) LE syndromes	Assess symptoms, history, fluid retention, posture, hormone changes, & circulatory compromise	Postural correction techniques Ergonomic assessment Splints for CTS

Adapted from Kisner C, Colby LA. *Therapeutic Exercise*, ed. 5. Philadelphia: FA Davis, 2007.

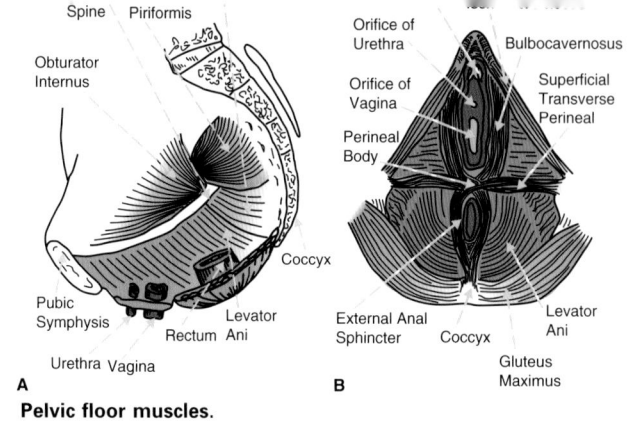

A

B

Pelvic floor muscles.

Kisner C, Colby LA. *Therapeutic Exercise*, ed. 5. Philadelphia: FA Davis, 2007.

Risk Factors for Pelvic Floor Dysfunction

- Childbirth, especially vaginal delivery
- Multiple deliveries
- Prolonged second stage of labor
- Use of forceps
- Use of oxytocin
- Perineal tears
- Birth weight >8 lb
- Chronic constipation
- Smoking
- Chronic cough
- Obesity
- Hysterectomy
- High caffeine intake*

*Risk factor for urge incontinence

Effect of Childbirth on Pelvic Floor

Impairments Induced During Childbirth	Outcome of Childbirth Impairments
Neurological compromise	Stretch & compression of pudendal nerve during labor as baby's head goes through canal (esp w/pushing)
Muscle impairment	Stretching during delivery & tears cause muscle weakness & dysfunction of pelvic floor musculature
Laceration during childbirth: episiotomy	No evidence to support use of episiotomy in labor & delivery.* Outcomes w/episiotomy are worse, including pain w/intercourse, extension of laceration to involve sphincter or rectum causing incontinence. Episiotomy does decrease fetal distress.

*Hartman, 2005.

Other Pelvic Floor Pathologies

Pathology	Description
Hypertonus dysfunction	↑ pelvic floor muscle tension/spasm causing pain/dysfunction in urogenital or colorectal
Cystocele	Herniation of urinary bladder into vagina
Rectocele	Herniation of rectum into posterior wall of vagina, causing a pouch in the intestine
Uterine prolapse	Bulging of uterus into vagina
Cystourethrocele	Bladder & urethra prolapse into vagina
Vaginal vault prolapse	Apex of vagina prolapses (sometimes after a hysterectomy)

Types	Definition	Causes
Stress (75% of all incontinence in women)	Incontinence when pressure ↑ to bladder, as from sneezing, laughing, exercising, coughing, or heavy lifts	Pelvic floor weakness Ligament or fascia laxity Urethral sphincter weakness **Risk factors:** pregnancy, vaginal delivery (long labor especially), heavy lifting, obesity, lack of hormone replacement in menopause, chronic constipation
Urge	Loss of urine when strong need to void (urgency)	Involuntary contraction of bladder Involuntary sphincter relaxation Alcohol, bladder infections, nerve damage, certain medications, interstitial cystitis
Mixed (combination urge & stress)	Combination of pressure & strong urge	Muscle weakness plus involuntary contraction of bladder or involuntary sphincter relaxation
Overflow	Overdistention of the bladder	A contractile bladder muscle Hypotonic/underactive bladder muscle due to drugs, fecal impaction, diabetes, lower SCI, or disruption of motor nerve of bladder muscle (in MS): results in urine retention & infection
		Men: mostly from prostate hyperplasia or carcinoma causing obstruction Women: severe genital prolapse or surgical overcorrection of urethral attachment causing obstruction
Bowel/bladder incontinence	Pressure or strong urge or gravity	Indication of SCI or nerve root damage

Common Symptoms of Perimenopause & Menopause

- Hot flashes, flushing, sweating
- Vaginal dryness, burning, itching
- Changes in body composition; especially weight gain
- Mood swings, irritability, depression
- Fatigue, headache, sleep disturbances
- Urinary incontinence, loss of pelvic muscle tone
- Decreased sexual drive
- Changes in bleeding and menstruation
- Tachycardia, heart palpitations
- Difficulty concentrating, memory issues

Effects of Menopause	
System	**Effects**
Musculoskeletal	↑ Bone loss, ↑ muscle injury, ↑ incidence of Colles fracture, carpal tunnel, osteoarthritis of basilar joint of thumb, rotator cuff limitation, & adhesive capsulitis
Connective tissue	Loss of collagen & elasticity
Muscle mass	↓ Levels of muscle mass w/↓ estrogen
Urogenital	Vaginal dryness, sexual dysfunction, & pain w/ intercourse

Cancers Found in Women

Cancer	Metastasis	Descriptions	Risk Factors	Signs & Symptoms
Breast	To lymph, bone, lung, brain, & liver	Most common cancers types: 1. Ductal CIS 2. Invasive (infiltrating) ductal CA (IDC) 3. Invasive infiltrating lobular 4. Medullary tubular & mucinous 5. Inflammatory breast 6. Paget disease of breast	Genetic mutation of BRCA1 & BRCA2 (10%) Fam Hx, early onset menstruation, infertility, age at first live birth > 35, high-dose radiation, high fat diet	Palpable lump or nodule that is firm & irregular Nodule found on mammogram One breast larger than other Local rash Discharge from nipple
Ovarian	To other organs	2nd most common female cancer, but highest mortality	Family Hx Personal Hx of endometrial or breast cancer at age 55–75 First birth later in life Positive BRCA1 or BRCA2 Obesity High-fat diet Prolonged exposure to estrogen	Usually none Abnormal bloating, discomfort, gastritis

Cancers Found in Women—cont'd

Cancer	Metastasis	Descriptions	Risk Factors	Signs & Symptoms
Cervical		Prevention w/regular pap smears	RFs: HPV virus, use of DES, smoking, hormonal contraceptive use, multiple births, young age at 1st intercourse, STDs	Often no symptoms May have spotty bleeding or pelvic pain
Endome-rrial/ uterine	To lymph	4th leading common cancer in women Women who exercise are 80% less likely to develop this cancer	Any condition that ↑ exposure to estrogen that is unopposed by progesterone	Abnormal bleeding

Diagnostic Test	Indications/Recommendations
Mammography	Reduces mortality from breast cancer by 20%–35% Recommendation is for mammography screening for breast cancer for women at age 40 & every 1–2 y after that
Digital mammography	Computerized x-rays that increase the likelihood of detection of masses
Ductal lavage	Insert microcatheter inside ductal glands inside nipple can identify cancer cells before mass or abnormal mammogram
Magnetic resonance imaging & PET scans	Help to stage breast cancer, but too costly to be used routinely. Cost effective for those already diagnosed w/breast cancer; used to screen for recurrence ACS guidelines recommend yearly MRI & mammo for high-risk females starting at age 30
Ultrasound	Used to differentiate a cyst from a solid lesion
Ultrasound elastography	Distinguishes harmless lumps from malignancies in minutes
Biomarkers	Protein C-ERBB-2 is a prognostic breast cancer marker found in biopsy specimens from those w/malignant tumors Tenascin-C also found in preinvasive & invasive cancer
Staging	Performed when all diagnostic test information is completed to determine optimal management of cancer Sentinel node biopsy to remove 1–3 nodes; >3 nodes removal is dissection

Interventions Used to Treat Women's Health Dysfunctions

Dysfunction	Possible Interventions
Pelvic floor prolapse Urinary incontinence	Pelvic floor rehabilitation including pelvic floor strengthening exercises (Kegels) Muscle re-education Postural education Biofeedback Electrical stimulation
Breast disease	Musculoskeletal strengthening & ROM if UE & lymph nodes involved Treatment for lymphedema including manual lymph drainage if necessary; compression garments, positioning are important
Menopause symptoms	Aerobic conditioning Decreasing fat from diet Alcohol & caffeine limitation

Practice Pattern	Includes Individuals With
Pattern 4B Impaired posture	Pregnancy-related changes Impaired joint mobility Inability to tolerate prolonged sitting Muscle weakness Mastectomy-related changes
Pattern 4C Impaired muscle performance	Pelvic floor dysfunction Stress urinary incontinence Diastasis recti Loss of muscle strength, power, endurance
Pattern 4D Impaired joint mobility, motor function, muscle performance, & ROM associated w/connective tissue dysfunction	Pregnancy-related strains/sprains Mastectomy-related muscle guarding, weakness, or lack of flexibility Ligamentous sprain Joint subluxation or dislocation Postpartum sacroiliac dysfunction Swelling or effusion Muscle guarding, weakness, or pain
Pattern 6H Impaired circulation & anthropometric dimensions associated w/ lymphatic system disorders	Lymphedema Reconstructive surgery Status post–lymph node dissection Post-radiation dysfunction

284

ICD 10 Codes Commonly Used With Pediatrics

P00–P96 Certain Conditions Originating in the Perinatal Period

P00–P04	Fetus and newborn affected by maternal factors and by complications of pregnancy, labor, and delivery
P05–P08	Disorders related to length of gestation and fetal growth
P10–P15	Birth trauma
P20–P29	Respiratory and cardiovascular disorders specific to the perinatal period
P35–P39	Infections specific to the perinatal period
P50–P61	Hemorrhagic and hematological disorders of fetus and newborn
P70–P74	Transitory endocrine and metabolic disorders specific to fetus and newborn
P75–P78	Digestive system disorders of fetus and newborn
P80–P83	Conditions involving the integument and temperature regulation of fetus and newborn
P90–P96	Other disorders originating in the perinatal period

Q00–Q99 Congenital Malformations, Deformations, and Chromosomal Abnormalities

Q00–Q07	Congenital malformations of the nervous system
Q10–Q18	Congenital malformations of eye, ear, face, and neck
Q20–Q28	Congenital malformations of the circulatory system
Q30–Q34	Congenital malformations of the respiratory system
Q35–Q37	Cleft lip and cleft palate
Q38–Q45	Other congenital malformations of the digestive system
Q50–Q56	Congenital malformations of genital organs
Q60–Q64	Congenital malformations of the urinary system
Q65–Q79	Congenital malformations and deformations of the musculoskeletal system
Q80–Q89	Other congenital malformations
Q90–Q99	Chromosomal abnormalities, not elsewhere classified

Past Medical History/Birth History
■ Significant medical history of biological parents
■ Mother's history during pregnancy, labor, and delivery
■ Child's history related to labor and delivery
■ Neonatal screening and immunization history
■ History of major childhood/adolescent illnesses
■ History of med/surgical procedures
■ Known allergies to food, medications, substances, etc

Developmental History
■ Infant/child temperament
■ Child/caregiver interactions & relationship
■ Growth and nutrition (grown chart)
■ Feeding: daily routine, preferences, or difficulties
■ Age of major milestone achievements
■ Bowel/bladder control and toilet training

Social History
■ Parents/caregivers' employment and hours working
■ Home layout, environment, exposures in home
■ Sleep routine of child
■ Use of car seat
■ School/daycare history
■ Signs of abuse or neglect

Apgar Scores				
	Signs	**0 Points**	**1 Point**	**2 Points**
A	Activity/muscle tone	Absent	Arms & legs flexed	Active movement
P	Pulse	Absent	Below 100 bpm	Above 100 bpm
G	Grimace (reflex irritability)	No response	Grimace	Sneeze, cough, pulls away
A	Appearance (skin color)	Blue-gray/pale all over	Normal except for extremities	Normal over entire body
R	Respiration	Absent	Slow, irregular	Good crying

Interpretation: ≥7 is normal, 4–6 fairly low, <4 critically low

Common Birth Defects

- Heart defects: 1/100
- Cleft lip/palate: 1/700. Possible speech, eating, & language problems
- Down syndrome: 1/800
- Spina bifida: 1 in 2500. Possible bowel/bladder problems or paralysis
- Other: musculoskeletal, gastrointestinal, metabolic

Common Birth Injuries

- **Bruising and forceps marks**
- **Caput succedaneum**—Severe swelling of the baby's scalp, as a result of vacuum extraction. Swelling disappears in a few days.
- **Cephalohematoma**—Bleeding between a bone and its fibrous covering on baby's head. Resolves within 2 weeks to 3 months.
- **Facial paralysis**—If nerve only bruised, it will clear in a few weeks. Severe damage may require surgery.
- **Brachial palsy injuries**—Erb palsy and Klumpke palsy.
- **Fractured bones**—Most common is to the clavicle (collar bone).
- **Brain injury**—Due to oxygen deprivation to the baby, and may result in seizure disorders, cerebral palsy, or mental impairment.

- **Bradypnea:** Respirations <30/min
- **Tachypnea:** Respirations >60/min
- **Abnormal breath sounds:** Crackles, wheezing, rhonchi, expiratory grunting
- **Respiratory distress:** Nasal flaring, retractions, labored breath, apnea

Oxygen Delivery

Modes: Oxygen tent/O_2 hood or incubator
Indications: For ↑ O_2 in peds settings; FIO_2 depends on incoming gas flow, volume of tent, degree tent is sealed
Limitations/constraints: Entering tent or hood alters the FIO_2; does not allow for much if any physical contact

Medical Diagnoses & Brief Descriptions

Diagnosis	Description
Arthrogryposis	↓ Fetal movements (akinesia), ↑ connective tissue around developing joints, contracture, abnormal muscle development
Asthma	Wheezing, coughing (nighttime & w/exercise), SOB, chest tightness, sputum production. Can be aggravated by allergens, irritants, exercise, & stress.
Cerebral palsy	Deficits in motor & postural control, sensory & perceptual function, communication & cognition that manifests in delayed motor development; Sz disorder common, often has cognitive & speech impairments, spasticity, & orthopedic issues
Congenital heart	Often present w/murmur, cyanosis of skin, lips, fingernails, & has SOB, fatigue, poor aerobic capacity

Diagnosis	Description
Cystic fibrosis	Genetic defect affecting respiratory & any other exocrine glands including pancreas & GI. Chronic respiratory infections & COPD, cough, airway obstruction, sputum, & GI & liver dysfunction. Requires digestive & pancreatic enzymes.
Development dysplasia of hip	Abnormal growth of hip, ↓ ROM, pseudoacetabulum, leg length difference, antalgic gait. Left side more often involved.
Down syndrome	Trisomy 21, facial characteristics, marked hypotonia, reduced reflexes, developmental delays, feeding problems, cardiac dysfunction, hip subluxation
Fetal alcohol syndrome	Low birth wt, failure to thrive, organ dysfunction, small head circumference, developmental delay, learning & cognitive difficulties (mental retardation, behavioral & social problems); skeletal & cardiac abnormalities may exist
Fractures: growth plate & long bone	Localized pain, swelling, unable to put wt on long bone. Growth plate fractures are concern for uneven growth.
Juvenile arthritis	Autoimmune disorder, with joint pain, stiffness, erythema, swelling, weakness, & decreased function & activity
Legg-Calve-Perthes	Limb with pain in hip, groin, thigh, or knee; ↓ ROM (internal rotation & abduction of hip)
Muscular dystrophy	Onset at birth or within 1st y; muscle dysfunction with variable presentation; hypotonia, feeding problems, spinal curvature, respiratory difficulties, cognitive or learning difficulties, Sz, cardiac & visual dysfunction
Neurofibromatosis	Tumors of any organ or system (most common: CNS, eyes, skin) that increase in number & size throughout life. Type 1 more skin & bone/joint less CNS tumors with improved prognosis. Type 2: meningiomas & acoustic neuromas.

Continued

Diagnosis	Description
Osteogenesis imperfecta	Hx of frequent fractures, ↓ bone density, bowing of long bones, bruising, blue sclera, short stature, dental & hearing & cardiac impairments
Scoliosis	Curvature of spine (>10°), postural asymmetries
Sickle cell anemia	Bouts of severe pain due to vaso-occlusive or aplastic crises, fatigue, ↓ resistance to infection, slow growth, delayed puberty. May develop cerebral infarction, pulmonary hypertension, renal failure.
Spina bifida	Motor & sensory loss due to failure of neural tube to close; foot deformities, hip deformities, hydrocephalus, neurogenic bladder
Torticollis	Unilateral tightening & shortening of sternocleidomastoid muscle, neck flexion to side of muscle involved, head rotation

Dole, 2010.

Children's Orientation & Amnesia Test (COAT) for Ages 3–15

Orientation Questions	Points Awarded	Max Score
What is your name?	2 = first name 3 = last name	5
How old are you? When is your birthday?	3 = correct age 1 = mo, 1 pt = y	5
Where do you live?	3 = city 2 = state	5
What is your father's name? What is your mother's name?	5 if either is correct	5
What school do you go to? What grade are you in?	3 2	5
Where are you now? OR Are you home now? Are you in a hospital?	5 Answer both for 5	5
Is it daytime or nighttime?	5	5
Total		35

Primitive Reflexes—Appearance & Timing

Reflex	Age (Months)							
	0	0.5	1	2	3	4	5	6
Suck/swallow								
Rooting								
Gallant								
Palmer grasp								
Plantar grasp								
Moro								
Stepping								

Attitudinal Reflexes—Appearance & Timing

Reflex	Age (Months)					
	2	4	6	8	10	12
ATNR						
TLR						
STNR						

Righting Reactions—Appearance & Timing

Reaction	Age (Months/Years)				
	2–3 mo	4–5 mo	1 y	5 y	Life
Optical					
Labyrinthine					
Body on head					
Landau					
Neck on body					
Body on body					

Protective Extension—Appearance & Timing

Reaction	Age (Months)				
	4–5	6–7	8–10	12–15	Life
Parachute LE					
Parachute UE					
Sitting to front					
Sitting to sides					
Sitting to back					
Standing					

Postural Fixation/Tilting Reactions—Appearance & Timing

Reaction	Age (Months)				
	5–6	7–8	9–10	12–15	Life
Prone					
Supine					
Sitting					
Quadruped					
Standing					

Adapted from Dole, **R**: *Peds Rehab Notes*. Philadelphia: FA Davis, 2010, p. 31.

Muscle Tone/Spasticity Assessment

Score	Spasm Frequency Scale
0	No spasms
1	Mild spasms induced by stimulation
2	Irregular strong spasms occurring <1/h
3	Spasms >1 h
4	Spasms >10/h

Adapted from Penn RD et al: Intrathecal baclofen for severe spinal spasticity. *N Engl J Med* 1989;320:1517.

Modified Ashworth Scale for Muscle Tone Assessment

Score	Description
0	No increase in muscle tone
1	Slight ↑ in muscle tone, observation of a catch & release or minimal resistance at end of ROM when part moved in flex/ext
1+	Slight ↑ in muscle tone, observation of a catch, minimal resistance throughout remainder of ROM
2	More marked ↑ in muscle tone through most of ROM but affected part easily moved
3	Considerable ↑ in muscle tone, passive movement difficult
4	Affected part rigid in flexion or extension

Adapted from Bohannon RW: Interrater reliability of a modified Ashworth scale of muscle spasticity. *Phys Ther*: 1987;67:207.

Neuromotor Development

Age	Gross Motor & Posture	Fine Motor	Cognitive
1 mo	Raises head while prone ABN reflexes present	Visual regard of objects Hands closed Swipes at objects	Scans within a face Shows preference for contrast
2 mo			Prefers normal face
3 mo	Rolls supine to side Rolls prone to supine accidentally	Glances from hand to object Reaches for but may not grasp object Visually directs reaching Hands clasped together often Sucking/swallow in sequence	
4 mo		Grasps rattle within 3 in Hands partially open	
5 mo	Rolls prone to supine segmentally	Holds objects Thumb opposition; attempts to pick up objects Grasps & draws bottle to mouth	Imitates new behavior
6 mo	Supports self in sitting Begins to go to quadruped position		Searches for completely hidden object Looks longer at scrambled face
7 mo	Crawls forward on belly Assumes quadruped position Begins pulling to stand at furniture Begins getting to sit from prone	Reaches w/one hand while prone	Engage in behaviors that produce specific effects. Repeat behaviors when wish to achieve same effect.

Continued

	Posture		
8 mo	Reciprocal creep on all fours Cruises sideways at furniture	Reaches & grasps	Purposefully carries out goal-directed behaviors
9 mo	Rises from supine by rolling to prone, pushing up to all fours	Feeds self crackers Holds bottle	Starts to learn that out-of-sight objects still exist
10 mo	Pulls to stand w/legs only Walks w/two hands held	Extends wrist, fingers Tries to feed self w/utensils	Explores cause & effect relationships & manipulates causes to achieve novel effects
11 mo	Takes independent steps Walking w/one hand held	Holds & drinks from cup Pincer grasp of finger foods	
12 mo	Rises to stand independently	Refines all fine motor skills from 12–24 mo:	
13 mo	Takes independent steps Lowers self from standing w/control Walking	Stacks blocks Turns pages Places toys in containers	
14–16 mo	Walks up stairs while holding on	Crayon held w/fist Covers/uncovers objects	Toddlers start to exhibit representational thoughts; internalize symbols as objects; use words for specific objects
17 mo	Walks down stairs while holding on	Turns knobs/handles Simple puzzles	
18 mo			

By age 2 children develop handedness (L vs. R) & by age 3 children may begin to demonstrate adult-like gait

Reflex Testing in Pediatric Patient/Clients

	Reflex	Stimulus	Response
Primitive/spinal	Flexor withdrawal	Pinprick to sole of foot in supine or sit position	Toes extend, foot dorsiflexes, leg flexes. Integrated 1–2 mo
	Crossed extension	Noxious stimulus to ball of foot while extremity in extension; patient/client supine	Opposite LE flexes, then adducts & extends. Integrated 1–2 mo
	Traction	Grasp forearm, pull up from supine to sit	Total flexion of UE. Onset 28 wk's gestation. Integrated 2–5 mo
	Moro	Sudden change in position of head	Extension, abduction of UE. Integrated 5–6 mo
	Startle	Sudden loud noise	Extension or abduction of arms. Persists through life
	Grasp	Pressure to palm of hand or ball of foot	Flexion of fingers or toes. Integrated 4–6 mo; fingers, 9 most toes
Tonic/Brain Stem	Asymmetrical tonic neck	Rotation of head to one side	Fencing posture: when face turned to one side, arm & leg of same side in extension, opposite side in flexion. Integrated 4–6 mo
	Symmetrical tonic neck	Flexion or extension of head	Flexion of head causes arm flexion, leg extension. With head extension: arm extension, leg flexion. Integrated 8–12 mo
	Symmetrical tonic labyrinthine	Prone or supine position	Prone: ↑ flexor tone. Supine: ↑ extensor tone. Integrated 6 mo
	Positive supporting	Pressure on ball of foot in stand position	Rigid extension of LE. Integrated 6 mo

Continued

	Reflex	Stimulus	Response
Tonic/Brain Stem	Associated reactions	Resisted voluntary movement in any part of body	Involuntary movement in resting extremity Integrated 8–9 y
	Neck righting action on the body	Passively turn head to one side while patient/client supine	Body rotation as a whole (log roll) Integrated 5 y
	Body righting acting on the body	Passively rotate upper or lower trunk segment	Body aligns w/rotated segment Integrated 5 y
	Labyrinthine head righting	Occlude vision, tip body in all positions	Head orients to vertical position Persists throughout life
	Optical righting	Alter body position by tipping in all directions	Head orients to vertical position Persists throughout life
	Body righting acting on body	Place prone or supine	Head orients to vertical Integrated 5 y
	Protective extension	Displace center of gravity outside base of support	Arms/legs extend & abduct to support & protect Persists throughout life
	Equilibrium reactions: tilting	Displace center of gravity by tilting or moving the support surface	Trunk curves toward upward side; extension & abduction of extremities on side; protective extension on opposite Persists throughout life
	Equilibrium reactions: postural fixation	Apply displacing force to body; alter center of gravity	Trunk curves toward external force w/extension & abduction of extremities on side force was applied Persists throughout life

Modified Glasgow Coma Scale for Infants & Children

Area Assessed	Infants	Children	Score*
Eye opening	Open spontaneously	Open spontaneously	4
	Open in response to verbal stimuli	Open in response to verbal stimuli	3
	Open in response to pain only	Open in response to pain only	2
	No response	No response	1
Verbal response	Coos & babbles	Oriented, appropriate	5
	Irritable cries	Confused	4
	Cries in response to pain	Inappropriate words	3
	Moans in response to pain	Incomprehensible words or nonspecific sounds	2
	No response	No response	1
Motor response†	Moves spontaneously & purposefully	Obeys commands	6
	Withdraws to touch	Localizes painful stimulus	5
	Withdraws in response to pain	Withdraws in response to pain	4
	Responds to pain with decorticate posturing (abnormal flexion)	Responds to pain with decorticate posturing (abnormal flexion)	3
	Responds to pain with decerebrate posturing (abnormal extension)	Responds to pain with decerebrate posturing (abnormal extension)	2
	No response	No response	1

*Score ≤12 suggests a severe head injury. Score <8 suggests need for intubation & ventilation. Score ≤6 suggests need for intracranial pressure monitoring.
†If the patient/client is intubated, unconscious, or preverbal, the most important part of this scale is motor response. This section should be carefully evaluated.
Adapted from Davis RJ et al: Head and spinal cord injury. In *Textbook of Pediatric Intensive Care*, edited by MC Rogers. Baltimore, Williams & Wilkins, 1987; James H, Anas N, Perkin RM: *Brain Insults in Infants and Children*. New York, Grune & Stratton, 1985; and Morray JP et al: Coma

Spectrum Disorders

Known Risk Factors	• Older sibling with autism • Diagnosis of tuberous sclerosis, fragile X, or epilepsy • A family Hx of autism or autistic-like behaviors
Warning Signs for Autism Screening	• No big smiles or other joyful expressions by 6 mo • No back-and-forth sharing of sounds, smiles, or facial expressions by 9 mo • No back-and-forth gestures, such as pointing, showing, reaching, or waving bye-bye by 12 mo • No babbling at 12 mo • No single words at 16 mo • No 2-word spontaneous (nonecholalic) phrases by 24 mo • Failure to attend to human voice by 24 mo • Failure to look at face & eyes of others by 24 mo • Failure to orient to name by 24 mo • Failure to demonstrate interest in other children by 24 mo • Failure to imitate by 24 mo • Any loss of any language or social skill at any age

Filipek et al., 1999; Greenspan, 1999; and Ozonoff, 2003.

Normal Pediatric Vital Signs

Age	Heart Rate		Respiratory Rate (breaths/min)
	Awake	Rest/Sleep	
Neonate	100–180	80–160	35–65
Infant	100–180	75–160	30–60
Toddler	80–110	60–90	24–40
Preschooler	70–110	60–90	22–34
School-age child	65–110	60–90	18–30
Adolescent	60–90	50–90	12–16

Blood Pressure (in mm Hg)

Age	Systolic	Diastolic
Birth at 12 h <1000 g	39–59	16–36
Birth at 12 hr 3 kg	50–70	25–45
Neonate at 96 h	60–90	20–60
Infant	87–105	53–66
Toddler	95–105	53–66
School-age child	97–112	57–71
Adolescent	112–128	66–80

Guide to PT Practice Patterns for Pediatric Populations

Pattern	Description
5B	Impaired Neuromotor Development
5C	Impaired Motor Function and Sensory Integrity Associated with Nonprogressive Disorders of the CNS—congenital Origin or Acquired in Infancy or Childhood
6G	Impaired Ventilation, Respiration/Gas Exchange and Aerobic Capacity Endurance Associated with Respiratory Failure in the Neonate

General Chemistry

Lab/NL Values	Deviations & Causes
Alanine aminotransferase (ALT) or SGPT 0–35 u/L	↑ in hepatitis, liver disease, bile duct damage, CHF, DM, mono, myopathy
Albumin/3.5– 5.5 g/100 mL	↓ in chronic liver disease; protein malnutrition, renal disease, malabsorption syndrome, chronic infection, acute stress
Aldolase/ 1.3–8.2 U/L	↑ in muscle or liver damage or disease
Alkaline phosphatase (ALP)/33–131 U/L Infants-adolescents <104 U/L Age >61 51–153	↑ in liver & bone diseases (obstructive & hepatocellular liver disease), obstructive jaundice, biliary cirrhosis, etc, ↑ in osteomalacia, metastatic bone disease & slight ↑ in healing fractures
Alpha-1 antitrypsin 1.5–3.5 g/L	↓ Indicates ↑ risk of panacinar emphysema at age <50 & liver cirrhosis
Ammonia/2–55 µmol/L	↑ in hepatic encephalopathy & Reye syndrome; tested to evaluate changes in consciousness
Amylase/30–100 U/mL	↑ in acute pancreatitis (first hs, NL in 2–3 d); ↑ for wks/mos w/chronic pancreatitis; ↑ in peritonitis, perforated peptic ulcer, acute intestinal obstruction, mesenteric thrombosis, & inflamm of salivary glands (e.g., mumps)
Anion gap/8–16 mEq/L	A calculated value using the results of electrolyte panel ↑ w/metabolic acidosis (e.g., uncontrolled DM, starvation, kidney damage, intake of toxic substances, ↑ aspirin, methanol) ↓ w/↓ albumin or w/↑ immunoglobulins

General Chemistry—cont'd

Lab/NL Values	Deviations & Causes
AST, SGOT <35 U/L	↑ in heart, liver, & skeletal muscle diseases & w/use of some meds ↑ in acute MI, necrosis of heart muscle (myocarditis), acute liver damage, cirrhosis, metastatic CA, obstructive jaundice, infectious mono, congestive hepatomegaly; ↑ in muscle diseases, gangrene of muscle, dermatomyositis, crush injury, & ingestion of aspirin, codeine, & cortisone
Bilirubin total/ <1.0 mg/100 mL	↑ w/destruction of RBCs: hemolytic diseases, hemorrhage, hepatic dysfunction, transfusion-initiated hemolysis, autoimmune disease
Brain natriuretic peptide BNP/<100 pg/mL	↑ w/heart failure <500 goal for hospital D/C >700 decompensated heart failure
BUN/8–22 mg/100 mL	↑ w/high protein intake, dehydration, burns, GI hemorrhage, renal disease, prostate hypertrophy ↓ w/low protein ingestion, starvation, liver dysfunction, cirrhosis
Calcitonin: ♀ 0–5 pg/mL ♂ 0–12 pg/mL	↑ in C-cell hyperplasia & MTC; used to screen for medullary thyroid cancer. Used to treat osteoporosis or hypercalcemia
Calcium/8.5– 10.5 mg/100 mL	↑ w/↑ vitamin D intake, osteoporosis, ↓ Na, ↓ urinary excretion, immobilization, ↑ Ca reabsorption, hypothyroidism ↓ w/↓ vitamin D intake, pregnancy, excessive diuretic, starvation ↓ Mg^{++}, acute pancreatitis, hypoalbuminemia
Carbon dioxide content/ bicarbonate or CO_2/24–30 mEq/L	Altered w/electrolyte imbalance; chronic disease, esp. kidney disease; & to evaluate acid-base balance; ↑ indicates alkalotic compensation or disease, ↓ in acidic compensation or metabolic acidosis

Continued

304

General Chemistry—cont'd

Lab/NL Values	Deviations & Causes
Chloride 95-105 mEq/L	↓ w/K+-sparing diuretics, vomiting, excess ↑ in K+ ingestion w/diarrhea, NH₄Cl ingestion (rarely)
Cholesterol/>200 mg/dL	↑ Indicates ↑ risk for heart disease
Cortisol/5-25 µg/ 100 mL (AM) <10 µg/100 mL (PM)	↑ in Addison disease & anterior pituitary hypofunction; ↓ Cushing syndrome & stress
Creatine/ ♂ 0.2-0.5 mg/ dL; ♀ 0.3-0.9 mg/dL	↑ in kidney disease/monitoring of progression of kidney function
Creatinine kinase <100 U/L	↑ in heart or skeletal muscle, progressive muscular dystrophy, cerebral infarcts
CK MB <5%	Isoenzymes distinguish origin of CPK ↑ (MM = skeletal muscle injury; MB ↑: cardiac muscle; BB ↑: brain injury)
Creatinine/0.6-1.3 mg/ 100 mL	↓ in renal disease/renal failure, chronic glomerulonephritis, hyperthyroidism; glomerular filtration rate (GFR) related to creatinine
C-reactive protein (CRP) <10 mg/L NL	10-40 mg/L mild inflamm or viral infection 40-200 mg/L bacterial infection
Ferritin: ♂ 10-400 ng/dL ♀ 10-200 ng/dL	↑ in chronic iron deficiency or if proteins are severely depleted, e.g., malnutrition ↓ in chronic iron excess (hemochromatosis)
Folate/2.0-9.0 ng/mL	↑ in vegan vegetarians & malnutrition, malabsorption as in celiac disease, Crohn disease, & cystic fibrosis; ↑ in pernicious anemia. ↑ stomach acid production, bacterial overgrowth in stomach, liver & kidney disease, alcoholism
Glucose/70-110 mg/100 mL	↓ in DM, pancreatic insufficiency, steroid use, pancreatic neoplasm, thiazide diuretics, excess catecholamines ↑ in beta cell neoplasm, hypothyroidism, starvation, glycogen storage diseases, Addison disease

General Chemistry—cont'd

Lab/NL Values	Deviations & Causes
Iron/50–150 µg/100 mL	↓ in anemia (as in chronic bleeding from gut or ↑ loss from heavy menstrual periods), chronic diseases such as cancers, autoimmune diseases, & chronic infections ↑ in hemochromatosis, excessive iron & heavy alcohol intake
Iron-binding capacity or transferrin/ 250–410 µg/ 100 mL	↑ in iron-deficiency anemia ↓ w/hemochromatosis, anemia from chronic infection or chronic disease, in liver disease (cirrhosis), & when ↓ protein in diet & in nephritic syndrome
Lactic acid (lactate) 6–16 mg/dL	↑ in hemorrhage, shock, sepsis, DKA, strenuous exercise, cirrhosis 2 × NL value found in severe sepsis
Lactic dehydrogenase (LDH)/45–190 U/L Has 5 isoenzymes	LDH1 ↑: MI, myocarditis, anemia, shock, malignancy LDH 2 ↑: MI, myocarditis, anemia, chronic granulocytic leukemia, pulmonary infarct, shock, malignancy LDH3 ↑: leukemia, pulmonary infarction, mononucleosis, shock, malignancy LDH4 ↑: mononucleosis, shock, malignancy LDH5 ↑: CHF, hepatitis, cirrhosis, skeletal muscle necrosis dermatomyositis, mononucleosis, shock, malignancy
Lipase/<200 U/mL	↑ in pancreatitis (very high) & kidney disease, salivary gland inflamm, & peptic ulcer; may be ↑ briefly w/tumor
Magnesium/ 1.5–2.0 mEq/L	↑ w/↑ ingestion of Mg^{++} (antacids) ↓ malabsorption syndrome, acute pancreatitis
Osmolality/ 280–296 mOsm/ kg H_2O	↑ w/dehydration ↓ w/fluid overload

Continued

General Chemistry—cont'd

Lab/NL Values	Deviations & Causes
Phosphate/3.0–4.5 mg/ 100 mL	↑ w/↑ growth hormone, chronic glomerulonephritis, sarcoidosis ↓ in hyperinsulinism, ↓ ingestion phosphorus
Potassium/ 3.5–5.0 mEq/L	↓ w/excess diuretic use, vomiting, cirrhosis, licorice intake, fasting/starvation ↑ in kidney disease, trauma, burns, excess replacement
Prealbumin/ 18–32 mg/dL	↓ poor nutrition/malnutrition Used to monitor treatment w/parenteral nutrition
Prostate-specific antigen/0–4.0 ng/mL	A tumor marker to screen for prostate cancer; ↑ in prostate cancer, prostatitis, & benign prostatic hyperplasia
Protein total/6.0–8.4 g /100 mL	Total protein alone is not informative unless albumin & globulin levels are known. ↓ liver or kidney disorder or when protein not absorbed; estrogen & oral contraceptives also ↓ protein.
Sodium/135–145 mEq/L	↓ in dehydration (burns, sweating, diarrhea), diuretics H_2O retention (CHF, renal, cirrhosis, excess intake), renal dysfunction, excess IV therapy ↑ w/excess H_2O loss, poor H_2O intake, hyperaldosteronism
T3/75–195 ng/100 mL	↓ hypothyroidism, rare pituitary hypothyroidism ↑ hyperthyroidism
T4 free/0.75–2.0 ng/dL	More accurate reflection of thyroid ↓ Hypothyroidism, rare pituitary hypothyroidism ↑ Hyperthyroidism

General Chemistry—cont'd

Lab/NL Values	Deviations & Causes
T4 total/4–12 μg/100 mL	Original test for thyroid function; now replaced w/free T4 ↓ in hypothyroidism, ↑ in hyperthyroidism
Thyroglobulin/ 3–42 μ/mL	Functions as tumor marker to assess effectiveness of thyroid cancer treatment & monitor recurrence; ↑ may indicate recurrence
Triglycerides/ 40–150 mg/ 100 mL	↑ in CAD, DM, nephritic syndrome, hepatic disease, & hypothyroidism
TSH/0.5–5.0 μ/mL	↑ indicates underactive thyroid, pituitary tumor, or lack of response to thyroid meds; ↓ indicates overactive thyroid or too much response to meds
Urea nitrogen/ 8–25 mg/100 mL	↑ in impaired kidney function from acute/chronic kidney disease or ↓ blood flow to kidneys (CHF, shock, MI, burns); also ↑ in excess protein breakdown or ↑ dietary protein or excess bleeding; ↓ liver disease, malnutrition, & overhydration
Uric acid/3.0–7.0 mg/100 mL	↑ in chronic lymphocytic & granulocytic leukemia, multiple myeloma, chronic renal failure, fasting, including ingestion of protein; gout, fasting, toxemia in pregnancy, ↑ salicylate ingestion, heavy alcohol intake

Rehabilitation Implications of General Chemistry

Abnormal Lab Test Result	Implications for Rehabilitation
↓ Albumin, ↓ prealbumin, ↓ protein	If malnourished, may have less energy for rehabilitation: poor exercise tolerance
↑ Cholesterol	Key risk factor for CVD; evaluate other risk factors & assess risk for CAD prior to exercise
↑ Creatine	May have ↓ kidney function
↑ Creatine kinase	May have muscle injury, including heart; check isoenzymes (BB, MB, MM)
↑ Creatinine	May have ↓ kidney function
↑ Glucose	May be prediabetic or diabetic: check fasting glucose, HbA1c
↓ Iron	↓ O_2 carrying capacity; ↓ endurance/exercise tolerance
↑ LDH	Check isoenzymes for organ dysfunction: liver? heart?
↑ Potassium	↑ Risk of arrhythmia, myocardial muscle contractility
↓ Potassium	↑ Risk of arrhythmia
↓ Sodium	Affects resting threshold of action potentials; may have leg cramping
↓ T4 free	May have ↑ wt; will have difficulty w/wt loss until T4 NL
↑ Uric acid	May have painful foot joint(s)/gout

Liver Function Tests

Lab/NL Values	Meaning of Abnormal Results
ALT/0–35 U/L	↑ Levels (10 × NL) w/acute hepatitis from acute infection & stay ↑ 1–3 mo ↑ in chronic hepatitis (4 × NL)
ALP/33–131 U/L	↑ Levels indicate bile duct blockage; if ALT & AST ↑, indicates ALP from liver; if ABN phosphorus & calcium, indicates ALP from bone
AST/0–35 U/L	↑ (10 × NL) w/acute hepatitis from acute viral infection, chronic hepatitis ↑ (4 × NL)
Bilirubin/ 0.3–1.0 mg/dL Newborn 1–12 mg/dL Critical: >15 mg/dL	↑ Too many RBCs destroyed or liver not removing bilirubin; ↑ in infants: kills brain cells & causes mental retardation; may occur w/RH incompatibility; ↑ in adults: metabolic problems, bile duct obstruction, damage to liver or inherited abnormality
Albumin/ 3.5–5 g/dL	↓ in liver & renal diseases, inflamm, shock & malnutrition; ↑ in dehydration
Total protein/ 7.0 g/dL	↓ in liver or kidney disorder or protein not being digested; ↓ albumin/globulin ratio in multiple myeloma or autoimmune diseases, cirrhosis or nephritic syndrome; ↑ in leukemia & genetic disorders

Hypertension Renal/Kidney Labs

Lab	NL Values	Rehabilitation Implications
BUN	8–25 mg/100 mL	↑ BUN in heart failure & renal failure; if ↑ creatinine, ↓ kidney functioning: indirect relationship between creatinine & GFR; ↑ creatinine means ↓ GFR
Creatinine	0.6–1.3 mg/100 mL	
Uric acid	3.0–7.0 mg/100 mL	

Cardiac Enzyme Markers

Lab/NL Values	Elevation Timetable	Rehabilitation Implications
Troponin I/0.0–0.4 ng/mL	↑ w/any cardiac muscle damage; tested 2–3× w/acute chest pain; remains ↑ 1–2 wk after MI	Elevated markers indicate acute myocardial injury; patient/client should be evaluated & treated for myocardial injury prior to rehab interventions; see note below w/ progression of values
Troponin T/<0.1 ng/mL		
CPK total <100 U/L	Begins to rise 2–12 h; returns to NL 2–4 d	
CPK-MB/<5%	Same as CK; also used to determine if clot-busting drugs working; will rise & fall faster w/drugs	
SGOT/AST <35 U/L	Begins to rise 6–24 h; returns to NL 3–6 d	
LDH/45–190 U/L	Begins to rise 12–48 h; returns to NL 7 d	
Myoglobin: ♂ 10–95 ng/mL; ♀ 10–65 ng/mL	Start to ↑ 2–3 h after MI, peak 8–12 h & returns to NL 24 h after	
C-reactive protein (CRP) <10 mg/L	↑ in acute inflamm Can indicate increased risk of CAD event Level of >2.4 mg/L indicates 2× coronary risk	

Cardiac Enzyme Markers: Progression Over Time

Marker	Onset	Peak	Duration
Troponin-I	3–6 h	12–24 h	4–6 d
Troponin-T	3–5 h	24 h	10–15 d
CPK	4–6 h	10–24 h	3–4 d
CPK-MB*	4–6 h	14–20 h	2–3 d
SGOT/AST	12–18 h	12–48 h	3–4 d
LDH	3–6 d	3–6 d	6–7 d
Myoglobin	2–4 h	6–10 h	12–36 h

Rehab Implications:
*Elevated markers indicate acute injury to myocardium; PK-MB must peak & start to ↓ before patient/client begins OOB activities & rehabilitation

Lipids

	NL Values	Deviations/Causes
Total cholesterol	<200 mg/dL adults 125–200 mg/dL child	↑ Values ↑ risk for developing CAD; must look at total HDL ratio
HDL	♂ >40 ♀ >50	↓ Values ↑ risk for developing CAD; must look at total HDL ratio
LDL	<100 mg/dL	↑ Values ↑ risk for developing CAD
VLDL	25%–50%	↑ Values ↑ risk for CAD & DM
Triglycerides	<150 mg/dL	↑ Values may ↑ risk for CAD & DM
Total/HDL ratio	<4:1 ratio	↑ Ratio ↑ risk for CAD
Lp(a)	<10 mg/dL	↑ Indicates ↑ risk for thrombosis & CAD
HbA1c	<6.5%	↑ % Indicates blood glucose has been out of NL range w/in last 3 mo; indicates control of blood sugars for 3 mo

Other Cardiovascular Tests

Test	NL Values	Deviations
Homocysteine	4–7 µmol/L	↑ Levels are a risk factor for CAD; ↑ in renal failure secondary to meds
C-reactive protein 1. High sensitivity CRP test for risk for CAD (cardio CRP) 2. Plain CRP test for inflamm or infection	<1.0 low CVD risk 1.0–3.0 average CVD risk 3.1–10 ↑ CVD risk	1. ↑ Levels near 10 mg/L associated w/↑ risk of atherosclerosis 2. ↑ Levels near 100 mg/L in noncoronary inflamm, infection
Brain natriuretic peptide (BNP)	<100 pg/mL	↑ w/heart failure <500 goal for hospital discharge >700 decompensated heart failure
Activated protein C resistance (APC-R)	<2.0 (ratio)	↑ Means ↑ for venous thromboembolic disease, CVD (♂ who smoke), & cerebrovascular disease; associated w/acute phase reactions ↑ risk in pregnancy
Verify now aspirin test (ARU = aspirin reaction units)	350–550 ARU = therapeutic range	>550 nontherapeutic range/ not reacting to aspirin

Coagulation Studies

Lab/NL Values	Deviations & Causes
ACT/175–225 sec	To monitor effect of high-dose heparin before, during, & after surgery ↑ = higher clotting inhibition (low platelets)
PTT or aPTT/ 20–35 sec Critical >100	Used for unexplained bleeding ↑ w/clotting problems, ↓ when coag factor VIII elevated or acute tissue inflamm/trauma
Bleeding time/ 1–9 min (IVY)*	↑ w/defective platelet function, thrombocytopenia, von Willebrand disease; also affected by drugs: dextran, indomethacin, & NSAIDs
Fibrinogen/ 150–400 mg/dL Critical <100	↑ in acute infections, coronary disease, stroke, MI, trauma, inflammatory disorders, breast/kidney/stomach cancer ↓ impairs ability to form clot, ↓ in liver disease, malnutrition, DIC, & cancers
INR/10–14 sec Critical >30	On anticoagulants: 2.0–3.0 for basic blood thinning, 2.5–3.5 for those w/higher clot risk (prosthetic heart valve, systemic emboli)
D dimer	Negative result: rules out VTE or low risk Positive test: requires further eval for VTE or PE
Plasminogen/ 80–92% of NL for plasma	The inactive form of plasminogen participates in fibrinolysis; used to evaluate hypercoagulable states (DIC, thrombus)
Platelets/ 150 K–450 K/mm†	Critical levels <50,000 or >999,000 ↑ inflammatory disorders & myeloproliferative states, hemolytic anemias, cirrhosis, iron deficiency, acute blood loss ↓ in aplastic anemia, megaloblastic & iron deficiency anemias, uremia, DIC, etc

Rehab Implications:
*Caution w/↑ bleeding time, ↑ PTT or aPTT; ↓ platelets: patient/client should not be falling, bumping, or bruising w/activity
†Critical level: platelets <50,000; may not be appropriate for rehab interventions

Lab Test	NL Values	Deviations/Causes
Blood volume	8.5–9.0% body wt (kg)	↓ Bleeding, burns, postsurgery
RBC × 10¹²/L	4.5–6.5 ♂ 3.9–5.6 ♀	↑ Polycythemia vera, chronic lung disease, dehydration, congenital heart disease, CVD, high altitude exposure, smoking history, renal cell CA ↓ Anemias, renal failure (chronic), SLE, leukemia, bone marrow dysfunction, Hodgkin disease, lymphomas, multiple myeloma, rheumatic fever
Hb (g/dL)	13.5–17.5 ♂ 11.5–15.5 ♀	↑ CHF, high altitude, dehydration, COPD ↓ Hemorrhage, anemia, cirrhosis, hemolysis
Hct (%)	40–52 ♂ 36–48 ♀	Same as Hb
Leukocytes (WBC) (× 10⁹/L)	4–11	Same as differentials
Bands	0%–5%	↓ Immunosuppressive meds, aplastic anemia, radiation to bone marrow, lymphocytic & monocytic leukemia, agranulocytosis, antibiotics, viral infections
Basophils	0%–1%	↑ Myelofibrosis, polycythemia vera, Hodgkin leukemia ↓ Anaphylactic reaction, stress, steroids, pregnancy, hyperthyroidism
Eosinophils	1%–4%	↑ Allergies (asthma, hay fever), parasites (roundworm, fluke), malignancy, colitis ↓ Burns, SLE, acute infection, mononucleosis, CHF, infections w/neutrophilia +/or neutropenia, meds (ACTH, thyroxine, epinephrine)

Hematology (CBC & blood counts)—cont'd

Lab Test	NL Values	Deviations/Causes
Lymphocytes • B-lymph • T-lymph	25%–40% 10%–20% 60%–80%	↑ Leukemia, infectious diseases, viral infections w/exanthema (measles, rubella); ↑ in viral infection, leukemia, bone marrow cancer, & radiation therapy; ↓ w/immune dysf (lupus & AIDS/HIV); ↑ in viral infection, leukemia, bone marrow cancer, & radiation therapy; ↓ w/immune dysf (lupus & AIDS/HIV)
Monocytes	2%–8%	↑ in viral diseases, neoplasms, inflammatory bowel, collagen diseases, hematology disorders
Neutrophils	54%–75%	> bacterial infections, inflammatory diseases, carcinoma, trauma, stress, corticosteroids, acute gout, DM, hemorrhage, hemolytic anemia; < acute viral infections, bone marrow disease, nutritional deficiency (vit B_{12}, folic acid)
Platelets ($\times 10^9$/L)	150–450	↓ in bone marrow disease (leukemia/thrombocytopenia), long-term bleeding problems, lupus, heparin or quinidine use, sulfa drugs, chemotherapy treatments ↑ in myeloproliferative disorders, living in high altitudes, strenuous exercise
ESR (mm/h)	1–13 ♂ 1–20 ♀	A nonspecific marker of inflamm; ↑ (excessively ↑) indicates acute infection; mod ↑ w/inflamm, anemia, infection, pregnancy, & ↑ age; ↑ in kidney failure, multiple myeloma, macroglobulinemia (tumors), & w/ oral contraceptives, theophylline, penicillin, & dextran; ↓ in polycythemia, leukocytosis, & some protein abnormalities; also ↓ w/aspirin, cortisone, & quinine

Rehab Implications:
• ↓ RBC or ↓ Hb: less O_2 carrying capacity/↓ exercise tolerance/endurance
• ↑ WBC indicates infection: VS may be abnormally ↑

Urinalysis

Lab	NL Findings	Deviations & Causes
Color/ appearance	Clear, yellow, straw	Lighter: urine diluted Dark: dehydration
Specific gravity	1.005–1.030	↓ Means urine diluted; ↑ means urine concentrated
pH	4.6–8.0	↓ Indicates acidosis, possibly secondary to ketones; ↑ Indicates alkalosis
Glucose	Negative	Abnormal blood sugars
Leukocyte esterase	Negative	Positive indicates urinary tract infection
Nitrite	Negative	Positive: urinary tract infection
Ketones	Negative	Positive: blood sugars out of balance
Protein	2–8 mg/dL	↑ Indicates ↓ renal function
Osmolality	300–900 mOsm/kg	Indicates diluted vs. concentrated urine ↑ Indicates dehydration, ↓ fluid overload
WBCs	3–4	↑ in urinary tract infection
RBCs	1–2	↑ w/damage to renal tubules
Crystals	Few/negative	↑ Indicates presence of renal stones
RBC or WBC casts	Negative	↑ w/upper urinary tract infections

CSF Analysis

Lab	NL Values
Pressure	50–180 mm H_2O
Appearance	Clear, colorless
Total protein	15–45 mg/dL
Prealbumin	2%–7%
Albumin	56%–76%
Alpha$_1$ globulin	2%–7%
Alpha$_2$ globulin	4%–12%
Beta globulin	8%–18%
Gamma globulin	3%–12%
Oligoclonal bands	None
IgG	<3.4 mg/dL
Glucose	500–800 mg/dL
Cell count	0–5 WBCs, no RBCs
Chloride	118–132 mEq/L
Lactate dehydrogenase	10% of serum level
Lactic acid	10–20 mg/dL
Cytology	No malignant cells
Culture	No growth
Gram stain*	Negative
India ink*	Negative
VDRL	Nonreactive

*Critical values: positive Gram stain, India ink prep, or culture

Med Levels (Therapeutic Levels/Toxic Levels)

Med	Therapeutic	Toxic
Acetaminophen	5–20 mg/L	>25 mg/L
Amiodarone	0.5–2.0 mg/L	>2.5 mg/L
Carbamazepine	4.0–12.0 µg/mL	>12
Digoxin/Lanoxin*	0.5–2.0 µg/L	2.2
Dilantin	10–20 µg/mL	>20
Lidocaine	1.5–5.0 mg/L	>7.0
Lithium	0.6–1.5 mEq/L	>1.5
Nitroprusside	<10 mg/dL	>10
Phenobarbital	15–40 µg/mL	>45
Procainamide	4–10 µg/mL	>15
Quinidine	1.2–4.0 µg/mL	>5.0
Salicylate	20–25 mg/100 mL	>30
Theophylline†	10–20 mg/L	>20

*Toxic levels Lanoxin: ↑ arrhythmias, changes on ECG, nausea
↑↑ Theophylline levels: therapeutic treatment not achieved for bronchodilation

Acid/Base Imbalances & Interpretation

	pH	pCO_2	HCO_2	Examples
Uncompensated respiratory acidosis	<7.35	>45	NL	Acute respiratory failure
Compensated respiratory acidosis	NL	>45	>26	Metabolically compensated respiratory failure
Uncompensated metabolic acidosis	<7.35	NL	<22	Diabetic ketoacidosis
Compensated metabolic acidosis	NL	<35	<22	
Acute respiratory alkalosis	>7.45	<35	NL	Hyperventilation, ↑ pain
Compensated respiratory alkalosis	NL	<35	<22	
Uncompensated metabolic alkalosis	>7.45	NL	>26	Nausea, vomiting
Fully compensated metabolic alkalosis	NL	>45	>26	

Arterial Blood Gases

Lab	NL Range	Possible Causes of Deviations
pH	7.35–7.45	↑ **(Alkalosis)** Metabolic: ↑ Ca++, overdose of alkaline substance, vomiting Respiratory: hyperventilation, pulmonary embolus ↓ **(Acidosis)** Metabolic: diarrhea, renal failure, aspirin overdose Respiratory: hypoventilation, respiratory depression, CNS depression
pO_2	75–100 mm Hg	↓ Values (hypoxia) in individuals w/lung disease, trauma, or infection; some interference w/O_2 getting into circulation; may require supplemental O_2
pCO_2	35–45 mm Hg	↓ Indicates hypocapnia: patient/client may be hyperventilating or blowing off too much CO_2 ↑ Indicates hypercapnia: patient/client retaining too much CO_2
HCO_3	22–26 mEq/L	↑ Levels indicate alkalosis: either a metabolic response to a respiratory acidosis or a primary metabolic disorder (e.g., vomiting) ↓ Indicates acidosis: either metabolic response to respiratory alkalosis or a primary metabolic disorder (e.g., diabetic ketoacidosis)
Base deficit/ excess	–2–+2 mEq/L	Reflects concentration of bicarbonate in body; >+3 or <–3 is critical
SpO_2	>95%	↓ Values indirectly indicate ↓ PO_2 in blood & O_2 dissociation; <90% critical; may require supplemental O_2

Index to More Commonly Used Medications

Drug	Classification
Actonel	Bone resorption blocker
Adderall	CNS stimulant
Advair	Inhaled steroid plus bronchodilator
Albuterol	Bronchodilator
Ambien	Sedative (sleep medicine)
Amiodarone	Anti-arrhythmia
Amlodipine (Norvasc)	Ca^{++} blocker
Aricept (donepezil)	Alzheimer
Atenolol (Tenormin)	Beta blocker
Altace (ramipril)	ACE inhibitor
Boniva	Bone resorption blocker
Calan (verapamil)	Ca^{++} blocker
Capoten	ACE inhibitor
Celebrex	NSAID
Cardizem (Diltiazem)	Ca++ blocker
Coreg (carvedilol)	Beta blocker
Coumadin	Anticoagulant
Dilantin	Antiseizure/convulsant
Diovan (valsartan)	Angiotensin renin blocker (ARB)
Dulera	Aerosol steroid plus bronchodilator
Exelon patch	Anti-Alzheimer
Lanoxin (digoxin)	Positive inotrope
Lantus	Long-acting insulin
Lasix	Diuretic
Lexapro	Antianxiety

Index to More Commonly Used Medications

Lipitor	Lipid lowering
Lisinopril (Prinivil)	ACE inhibitor
Lortab	Pain med
Lovenox	Anticoagulant
Lunesta	Sedative
Lyrica	Anticonvulsant
Namenda (memantine)	Anti-Alzheimer
Naproxen (Naprosyn)	NSAID
Niaspan	↑ HDL
Nitroglycerine	Nitrate: anti-angina
Norvasc (amlodipine)	Ca^{++} blocker
Oxycontin	Pain med
Paxil	Anti-anxiety/antidepressant
Percocet	Pain med
Phenergan	Sedative/antianxiety
Plavix	Antiplatelet
Prednisone	Steroid: Anti-inflammatory
Spiriva	Bronchodilator
Toprol (metoprolol)	Beta blocker
Tramadol	Pain med
Vytorin (Zetia & Zocor)	Lipid-lowering
Xopinex	Bronchodilator
Zocor	Lipid-lowering

Traditional Medications

Anti-Alzheimer

Caprylidene (Axona) Donepezil (Aricept) Galantamine (Reminyl) Memantine (Namenda) Rivastigmine (Exelon) Tacrine (Cognex)	**Indications:** Management of dementia **Effect:** ↑ Amount of acetylcholine in CNS (inhibits cholinesterase); temperature ↑ cognitive function & QOL **Common side effects:** Fatigue, dizziness, HA, diarrhea, nausea, incontinence, tremor, arthritis, muscle cramps **Contraind:** Hypersensitivity **Use cautiously:** W/hepatic reaction

Antianemics

Anadrol Chromagen Cyanocobalamin Hydroxocobalamin (vit B_{12} prep) Folic acid Darbepoetin Epoetin (Procrit) Nandrolone (Decan) Carbonyl iron (Feosol) Ferracon Ferrex 150 Ferrous fumarate (Femiron) Ferrous gluconate Ferrous sulfate (Slow Fe) Ferumoxytol (Feraheme) Integra Iron (Dextran)	**Indications:** Prevention & treatment of anemias **Effect:** RBC & Hb production **Common side effects:** 1. Oral Fe ↓ absorption of tetracyclines 2. Vit E ↓ response to Fe 3. Phenytoin (anticonvulsant) ↓ absorption of folic acid 4. Darbepoetin & epoetin may ↑ heparin need in hemodialysis **Other side effects:** Dizziness, HA, nausea, vomiting **Contraind:** All are contraind in undiagnosed anemias, uncontrolled HTN, hemolytic anemias **Use cautiously:** Use parenteral iron cautiously in patient/clients w/ hypersensitive reactions or allergies

Antianginals

Nitrates Isosorbide dinitrate Isordil Nitroglycerin **Beta Blockers**	**Nitrates** **Indications:** Treat & prevent angina attacks & acute angina **Effect:** Dilate coronary arteries; cause systemic vasodilation

Continued

Atenolol (Tenormin) Carteolol (Cartrol) Carvedilol (Coreg) Labetalol (Normodyne) Metoprolol (Toprol, Lopressor) Nadolol (Corgard) **Ca⁺ Channel Blockers** Amlodipine (Norvasc) Bepridil (Vascor) Diltiazem (Cardizem) Verapamil (Calan, Isoptin)	**Common side effects:** Nitrates cause headaches; need to develop tolerance **Ca+ Channel Blockers & Beta Blockers** **Indications:** Long-term management of angina **Effect:** *Beta blockers* ↓ Myocardial O₂ consumption: ↓ HR **Ca⁺ Channel Blockers** Smooth muscle arterial relaxation (systemic) **Common side effects:** Hypotension/dizziness, particularly w/position changes (orthostatic hypotension) **Contraind/cautions:** Beta blockers & Ca⁺ channel blockers: contraind in advanced heart block, cardiogenic shock, & uncomp heart failure

Antianxiety

Benzodiazepines Alprazolam (Xanax) Chlordiazepoxide (Librium) Clonazepam (Klonopin) Diazepam (Valium) Escitalopram (Lexapro) Lorazepam (Ativan) Midazolam (Versed) Oxazepam (Serax)	**Indications:** Management of anxiety: general anxiety disorder; short-term: benzodiazepines; long-term: buspirone, paroxetine, venlafaxine **Effect:** Generalized CNS depression; benzodiazepine: psychological or physical dependence
Others Buspirone (BuSpar) Desvenlafaxine (Pristiq) Doxepin (Sinequan) Gabapentin (Neurontin) Hydroxyzine (Atarax/Vistaril) Mirtazapine (Remeron) Oxcarbazepine (Trileptal) Paroxetine (Paxil) Prochlorperazine (Compazine) Venlafaxine (Effexor)	**Common side effects:** May cause daytime drowsiness; avoid driving & other activities requiring alertness **Others:** dizziness, lethargy, blurred vision, hypotension, physical dependence on meds **Contraind:** Do not use if pregnant or breastfeeding Not used w/uncontrolled severe pain **Cautions:** Avoid alcohol & other CNS depressants

Antiarrhythmics

Class IA Disopyramide (Norpace) Moricizine (Ethmozine) Procainamide (Procan) Quinidine **Class 1B** Lidocaine Mexiletine (Mexitil) Phenytoin (Dilantin) Tocainide (Tonocard) **Class 1C** Flecainide (Tambocor) Propafenone (Rythmol) **Class II** Acebutolol (Sectral) Esmolol (Brevibloc) Propranolol (Inderal) Sotalol (Betapace)	**Indications:** Suppress cardiac arrhythmias Goal: ↓ Symptoms & ↑ hemodynamic performance Classified by effect on cardiac conduct tissue **Effect: Class IA:** ↓ Na^{++} conduction, ↑ action potential & effective refraction period, ↓ membrane response **Effect: Class IB:** ↑ $K+$ conduction, ↓ action potential duration & refractory period **Class IC:** Slow conduction, ↓ phase 0 **Class III:** Interferes with Na conduction, depresses cell membrane, ↓ automaticity, blocks ↑ symptom activity **Class III:** Interferes w/norepinephrine, ↑ AP & refractory period **Class IV:** ↑ AV nodal refractory period; calcium channel blocker
Class III Amiodarone (Cordarone, Pacerone) Dofetilide (Tikosyn) Ibutilide (Corvert) **Class IV** Diltiazem (Cardizem) Verapamil Multaq (Dronedarone) **Others** Adenosine Atropine Digoxin	**Common side effects:** Dizziness, fatigue, headache, nausea, constipation, dry mouth, hypotension, ↑ arrhythmias, s/s of heart failure, hypoglycemia, fever **Contraind:** NOT used in individuals w/ second- or third-degree heart block or in cardiogenic shock **Caution:** Take apical pulse before administering oral doses (no <50 bpm)

Antiasthmatics

Bronchodilators Albuterol (Proventil) Epinephrine Formoterol (Foradil) Levalbuterol (Xopenex)	**Indications:** Management of acute & chronic episodes of reversible bronchoconstriction Goal: treat acute attacks & ↓ incidence & intensity of future attacks

Continued

Metaproterenol (Alupent)
Pirbuterol (Maxair)
Salmeterol (Serevent)
Terbutaline (Brethaire)
Corticosteroids
Beclomethasone (Beclovent,
  Vanceril)
Betamethasone
Budesonide (Pulmicort)
Cortisone
Dexamethasone (Decadron)
Flunisolide (Aerobid)
Fluticasone (Flovent)
Hydrocortisone
Methylprednisolone
Prednisone
Triamcinolone (Azmacort)
Combination
Advair (bronchodilator &
  steroid inhaled)
Combivent (two
  bronchodilators)
Dulera (bronchodilator &
  steroid)
Leukotriene Receptor
Antagonist
Zafirlukast (Accolate)
Montelukast (Singulair)
Mast Cell Stabilizers
Cromolyn
Nedocromil (Tilade)
	Effect: Bronchodilators &
	phosphodiesterase inhibitors act on
	intracellular cycles 3, 5 AMP by ↓
	production or ↓ breakdown;
	corticosteroids ↓ airway inflammation;
	leukotriene receptor antagonists ↓
	substances that induce bronchoconstriction
	Common side effects: Nervousness,
	restlessness, tremors, insomnias,
	palpitations, hyperglycemia, arrhythmias
	Corticosteroids: Depression, euphoria,
	personality changes, HTN, peptic
	ulceration, ↓ wound healing, wt gain,
	cushingoid appearance
	Contraind/cautions: Long-acting
	adrenergics, mast cell stabilizers, &
	inhaled corticosteroids: NOT used during
	acute attacks
	Caution: Adrenergics & anticholinergics
	w/CVD
	Corticosteroids: Should NOT be stopped
	abruptly; long-term use of systemic
	corticosteroids may ↓ bone & muscle
	mass & ↑ glycemic control

Anticholinergics	
Atropine Benztropine Biperidin Glycopyrrolate Ipratropium (Atrovent) Oxybutynin Propantheline Scopolamine Tiatropium (Spiriva)	**Indications:** Bradyarrhythmias, bronchospasm, nausea & vomiting from motion sickness, ↓ gastric secretory activity, used for Parkinson disease **Effect:** Inhibit acetylcholine & action of acetylcholine at sites innervated by postganglionic cholinergic nerves **Common side effects:** Drowsiness, dry mouth, dry eyes, blurred vision,

Tolterodine Trihexyphenidyl	constipation, inhibits absorption of other drugs; alters GI motility & transit time **Contraind:** Geriatric & pediatric patient/clients more prone to adverse effects **Use cautiously:** W/chronic renal, hepatic, pulmonary, or cardiac disease

Anticoagulants

Coumadin (warfarin) Fondaparinux (Arixtra) Dalteparin (Fragmin) Danaparoid (Orgaran) Enoxaparin (Lovenox) Tinzaparin (Innohep) Argatroban Bivalirudin (Angiomax) Lepirudin (Refluden) ATryn (antithrombin recombinant) Effient (Prasugrel) **Specific for Atrial Fib** Pradaxa Xarelto Eliquis (Apixaban)	**Indications:** Prevent & treat thromboembolic disorders: pulmonary emboli, atrial fibrillation, phlebitis Used for mgmt of MI **Effect:** Prevent clot formation & extension; heparin used first: rapid onset of action, followed by maintenance therapy **Common side effects:** Dizziness, bleeding, anemia, thrombocytopenia **Contraind:** NOT indicated for coagulation disorders, ulcers, malignancies, recent surgery, or active bleeding. **Use cautiously:** W/patient/clients at risk for ↑ bleeding

Anticonvulsants

Barbiturates Pentobarbital Phenobarbital **Benzodiazepines** Diazepam **Other** Acetazolamide Carbamazepine Divalproex sodium Gabapentin (Neurontin) Lacosamide (Vimpat) Phenytoin (Dilantin) Pregabalin (Lyrica) Valproate sodium Vigabatrin (Sabril) Zonisamide	**Indications:** ↓ Incidence & severity of seizures **Effect:** ↓ Abnormal neuronal discharges in CNS; raise seizure threshold, alter levels of neurotransmitters, ↓ motor cortex, or prevent spread of seizure activity **Common side effects:** Ataxia, agitation, nystagmus, diplopia, HTN, nausea, altered taste, anorexia, agranulocytosis, aplastic anemia, fever, rashes, hangover, nausea, hypotension **Use cautiously:** W/severe hepatic or renal disease & w/pregnant females or breastfeeding mothers

Continued

Antidepressants

MAO Inhibitors
Phenelzine (Nardil)
Tranylcypromine (Parnate)
Serotonin Reuptake Inhibitors
Citalopram (Celexa)
Duloxetine (Cymbalta)
Fluoxetine (Prozac)
Fluvoxamine (Luvox)
Paroxetine(Paxil)
Sertraline (Zoloft)
Tricyclics
Amitriptyline (Elavil)
Amoxapine
Desipramine
Doxepin (Sinequan)
Imipramine (Tofranil)
Nortriptyline (Pamelor)
Others
Mirtazapine (Remeron)
Bupropion (Wellbutrin or Aplenzin)
Nefazodone
Trazodone (Oleptro)
Venlafaxine (Effexor)

Indications: Depression
Anxiety (doxepin); enuresis (imipramine), chronic pain (amitriptyline, doxepin, imipramine, nortriptyline); smoking cessation (bupropion); bulimia (fluoxetine); obsessive-compulsive disorder (fluoxetine, sertraline); & generalized anxiety (venlafaxine, paroxetine)
Effect: Prevent reuptake of dopamine, norepinephrine, & serotonin by presynaptic neurons
Result: Accumulation of neurotransmitters. Most tricyclics: anticholinergic & sedative properties
Common side effects: Drowsiness, insomnia, dry eyes, dry mouth, blurred vision, constipation, orthostatic hypotension, dizziness
Contraind: Hypersensitivity, glaucoma, pregnancy, lactation, immediate post MI.
Use cautiously: W/elderly patient/clients w/preexisting CAD, prostate enlargement, slow titration

Antidiabetics

Acarbose (precose)
Cycloset (bromocriptine)
Glimepiride (Amaryl)
Glipizide (Glucotrol)
Glyburide (micronase)
Insulin
Lantus (Long-acting)
Liraglutide (Victoza)
Metformin (glucophage)
Miglitol (Glyset)

Indications: Management of DM to control (lower) blood sugar; PTs should know time of onset and time of peak effect of these meds
Effect: Lower blood sugar
Common side effects: Hypoglycemia. Dosage altered frequently due to stress, infection, exercise, changes in diet, etc
Contraind: Hypoglycemia, hypersensitivity, infection, stress, or changes in diet may alter dosage
Use cautiously: W/elderly patient/clients

Nateglinide (Starlix) NPH insulin Saxagliptin (Onglyza) Pioglitazone (Actos) Repaglinide (Prandin) Liraglutide (Victoza)	
Antifungals	
Amphotericin Caspofungin Fluconazole Griseofulvin Itraconazole Ketoconazole Terbinafine	**Indications:** Treatment of fungal infections **Effect:** Kill/stop growth of susceptible fungi: affects permeability of fungal cell membrane or protein synthesis **Common side effects:** Skin irritation ↑ Risk of infection **Use cautiously:** Patient/clients w/↓ bone marrow function. May ↓ bone marrow function
Antihistamines	
Azatadine Brompheniramine Cetirizine (Zyrtec) Chlorpheniramine (Chlor-Trimeton) Cyproheptadine (Periactin) Desloratidine Hydroxyzine (Vistaril) Loratadine (Claritan) Olopatadine hydrochloride (Patanase) Promethazine (Phenergan)	**Indications:** Relief of allergy symptoms (rhinitis, urticaria, angioedema) Also used as adjunctive therapy in anaphylactic reactions **Effect:** Block effect of histamine at H1 receptor **Common side effects:** Constipation, dry mouth, dry eyes, blurred vision, sedation **Contraind:** Hypersensitivity, narrow-angle glaucoma, prematurely born infants or newborns. **Use cautiously:** W/elderly, pyloric obstruction, prostate hypertrophy, hyperthyroidism, cardiovascular & liver disease.

Continued

Antihypertensives

ACE Inhibitors Benazepril Captopril Enalapril Fosinopril Lisinopril Moexipril Perindopril Quinapril Ramipril (Altace) Trandolapril	**Indications:** Treatment of ↑ BP & management of CHF/slows progression of L ventricle dysfunction Lisinopril: used in prevention of migraines **Effect:** Lower BP, ↓ afterload in CHF, ↓ development of overt HF, ↑ survival after MI, blocks angiotensin I → vasoconstriction angiotension II Activates vasodilation bradykinins **Common side effects:** Dizziness, fatigue, HA, rash, insomnia, angina, weakness, **cough,** hypotension, taste disturbance, cough, proteinuria, impotence, nausea, hyperkalemia, anorexia, diarrhea, neutropenia **Contraind:** Hypersensitivity, pregnancy, angioedema. **Use cautiously:** W/renal or hepatic impairment, hypovolemia Concurrent diuretic therapy, elderly, aortic stenosis, cerebrovascular or cardiac insufficiency, family Hx of angioedema
Angiotensin II Receptor antagonists Candesartan Eprosartan Irbesartan Losartan Telmisartan Valsartan (Diovan)	**Indications:** Management of HTN **Effect:** ↓ BP; blocks vasoconstriction effects of angiotension II at receptor sites: smooth muscle & adrenal glands **Common side effects:** Dizziness, fatigue, HA, hypotension, diarrhea, drug-induced hepatitis, renal failure, hyperkalemia **Contraind:** Hypersensitivity, pregnancy or lactation. **Use cautiously:** W/CHF, volume- or salt-depleted patient/clients, patient/clients w/diuretics, impaired renal, obstructive biliary disorders, age <18 y.

Beta Blockers: Nonselective Carteolol Carvedilol Labetalol Nadolol Penbutolol Pindolol Propanolol Timolol	**Indications:** Management of: HTN & angina, may be used for prevention of MI **Effect:** Overall: ↓ HR & RP **Nonselective:** Blocks stimulation of both beta-1 & beta-2 adrenergic recap sites **Selective:** Blocks stimulation of beta-1 receptors; no effect on beta-2 receptors
Beta Blockers: Selective Acebutolol Atenolol Betaxolol Bisoprolol Metoprolol	**Common side effects:** Fatigue, weakness, impotence, anxiety, depression, mental status changes, memory loss, dizziness, drowsiness, insomnia, blurred vision, nervousness, nightmares, CHF, bronchospasm (nonselective), bradycardia, hypotension, peripheral vasoconstriction, hyper- & hypoglycemia, GI disturbance **Contraind:** Uncomp CHF, pulmonary edema, cardiogenic shock, bradycardia or heart block. **Use cautiously:** W/renal or hepatic impairment, geriatric patient/clients, pulmonary disease, diabetes, thyrotoxicosis, allergic reactions, & pregnancy.
Calcium Channel **Blockers** Amlodipine (Norvasc) **Clevidipine** (IV only) Diltiazem (Cardizem) Felodipine Isradipine Nicardipine Nifedipine (Procardia) Nisoldipine Verapamil (Calan/Isoptin)	**Indications:** Management of HTN disease, angina pectoris, & vasospastic (Prinzmetal angina) **Effect:** Systemic vasodilation: w/↓ BP, coronary vasodilation: ↓ frequency & attacks of angina. Inhibits transport of Ca++ → myocardial & vascular smooth muscle cells **Common side effects:** HA, peripheral edema, dizziness, fatigue, angina, bradycardia, hypotension, palpitations, flushing, nausea

Continued

	Contraind: Hypersensitivity & BP <90 mm Hg, bradycardia, second- or third-degree block or uncomp CHF: **Use cautiously:** W/severe hepatic impairment, geriatric patient/clients, aortic stenosis, Hx of CHF, pregnancy, lactation, or children
Diuretics Chlorothiazide (Diuril) Chlorthalidone (Hygroton) Furosemide (Lasix) Hydrochlorothiazide (HydroDiuril) Indapamide Metolazone	**Indications:** Management of HTN or edema due to CHF or other causes; potassium-sparing diuretics have weak antihypertensive properties; used to conserve K+ **Effect:** ↑ excretion of electrolytes & H_2O working on renal system **Common side effects:** Hypokalemia, hyperuricemia, dizziness, lethargy, weakness, ↓ BP, anorexia, cramping, hyperglycemia, dehydration, hyponatremia, muscle cramps, pancreatitis **Contraind:** Hypersensitivity. **Use cautiously:** W/renal or hepatic disease
Others Clonidine Doxazosin Fenoldopam Guanabenz Guanadrel Guanfacine Methyldopa Minoxidil Nitroprusside Prazosin Terazosin	**Indications:** Treatment of essential HTN; therapy initiated w/agents w/minimum side effects, w/more potent drugs added to control BP **Effect:** To ↓ diastolic BP to <90 mm Hg or to lowest tolerated level Antiadrenergic properties (peripheral & central) & vasodilation **Common side effects:** Dizziness, hypotension, weakness, dry mouth, bradycardia, sodium retention, GI problems **Use cautiously:** W/renal dysfunction & uncompensated CHF

Antibiotics	
Aminoglycosides (antibiotics) Gentamicin Kanamycin Neomycin Streptomycin Tobramycin **Cephalosporins** Cefadroxil (Duricef) Cefazolin (Ancef) Cefuroxime (Ceftin) Cephalexin (Keflex) **Fluoroquinolones** Ciprofloxacin (Cipro) Enoxacin (Penetrex) Gatifloxacin (Tequin) Levofloxacin (Levaquin) **Macrolides** Azithromycin (Zithromax) Clarithromycin (Biaxin) Erythromycin **Penicillins** Amoxicillin (Amoxil) Ampicillin **Sulfonamides** Sulfacetamide Sulfamethoxazole **Tetracyclines** Ceftaroline fosamil (Teflaro) Doxycycline Minocycline Tetracycline **Others** Cloxacillin (Cloxapen) Dicloxacillin (Dycill) Nafcillin (Nallpen) Vancomycin	**Indications:** Treat/prevent bacterial infections **Effect:** Kill/inhibit growth of pathogenic bacteria; do not work against fungi or viruses **Common side effects:** Diarrhea, nausea, vomiting, rashes, urticaria, seizures, dizziness, drowsiness, HA **Contraind:** W/hypersensitivity to specific drugs. **Use cautiously:** W/pregnant or lactating women, hepatic or renal insufficiency Prolonged use of broad-spectrum drugs may lead to additional infection w/fungi or resistant bacteria.

Continued

Antineoplasms

Alkylating Agents Busulfan Chlorambucil Melphalan Procarbazine **Anthracyclines** Doxorubicin Epirubicin **Antitumor Antibiotic** Bleomycin Mitomycin **Hormonal Agents** Estramustine Letrozole Tamoxifen **Vinca Alkaloids** Vinblastine Vincristine OTHER: Sancuso (granisetron) Arzerra (ofatumumab) Folotyn (pralatrexate) Isodax (romidepsin) Afinitor (everolimus) Avastin (bevacizumab) Jevtana (cabazitaxel) Provenge (sipuleucel-T) Halaven (eribulin mesylate) Xgeva (denosumab) Mozobil (plerixafor) Degarelix Treanda Herceptin (trastuzumab)	**Indications:** Treatment of solid tumors, lymphomas, & leukemias; often combine meds **Effect:** Various agents have various effects; may affect DNA synthesis or function, alter immune function or hormonal status; may affect other cells besides neoplastic cells **Common side effects:** Nausea, vomiting, alopecia, anemia, leukopenia, thrombocytopenia, GI disturbances, pulmonary fibrosis, itching, rashes, arthralgia, myalgia, chills, fever, infection, hot flashes **Contraind:** Previous bone marrow depression or hypersensitivity, pregnancy, or lactation. **Use cautiously:** Patient/clients w/active infections, ↓ bone marrow reserve, radiation therapy, or debilitating illness

Antiparkinson Agents

Benztropine Biperiden Bromocriptine Carbidopa	**Indications:** Treatment of Parkinson disease of various causes: degenerative, toxic, infective, neoplastic, or drug-induced

Entacapone Levodopa Pergolide Pramipexole Ropinirole Selegiline	**Effect:** Reduction of rigidity & tremors; restores balance of major neurotransmitters: acetylcholine & dopamine; ↓ dopamine results in ↑↑ cholinergic activity **Common side effects:** Blurred vision, dry eyes, dry mouth, constipation, confusion, depression, dizziness, HA, sedation, weakness **Contraind:** Patient/clients w/narrow-angle glaucoma. **Use cautiously:** W/severe cardiac disease, pyloric obstruction, or prostate enlargements

Antiplatelets

Aspirin Cilostazol Clopidogrel (Plavix) Dipyridamole (Persantine) Eptifibatide (Integrilin) Ticlopidine (Ticlid) Tirofiban (Aggrastat)	**Indications:** Treatment & prevention of thromboembolic events (stroke, MI) Dipyridamole used after cardiac surgery **Effect:** Inhibit platelet aggregation Some inhibit phosphodiesterase **Common side effects:** HA, dizziness, hypotension, palpitations, tachycardia, nausea, diarrhea, gastritis, GI bleeding **Contraind:** Hypersensitivity, ulcer disease, active bleeding, recent surgery. **Use cautiously:** In patient/clients at risk for bleeding (surgery or trauma), Hx of GI bleeding or ulcers

Antipsychotics

Chlorpromazine Clozapine Fluphenazine Haloperidol (Haldol) Olanzapine (Zyprexa) Prochlorperazine (Compazine) Quetiapine (Seroquel)	**Indications:** Treatment of psychoses: acute & chronic; treatment of psychomotor activity associated w/psychoses **Effect:** Decrease S & S of psychoses; block dopamine receptors in brain; alter dopamine release & turnover Anticholinergic effects peripherally

Continued

Risperidone Thioridazine (Mellaril) Trifluoperazine Ziprasidone (Geodon)	**Common side effects:** Extrapyramidal reactions, dyskinesia, sedation, photosensitivity, blurred vision, dry eyes, dry mouth, leukopenia, constipation, hypotension **Contraind:** Hypersensitivity, w/narrow-angle glaucoma, & w/CNS depression. **Use cautiously:** W/CAD; severely ill, debilitated patient/clients; diabetics, w/ respiratory insufficiency, hypertrophy of prostate, intestinal obstruction
Antirheumatics	
Corticosteroids Betamethasone Cortisone Dexamethasone Hydrocortisone Methylprednisolone Prednisone **Disease-Modifying Antirheumatics (DMARDs)** Anakinra Azathioprine (Imuran) Etanercept Hydroxychloroquine Infliximab Leflunomide Methotrexate Pencillamine **NSAIDs** See below under **NSAIDs**	**Indications:** Management of pain & swelling in RA, ↓ progression of disease, & joint destruction; preserve joint function **Effect:** NSAIDs & corticosteroids are anti-inflammatory meds; DMARDs suppress autoimmune response (cell-mediated immunity & altered antibody formation) **Common side effects:** Steroids: depression, nausea, euphoria, anorexia, HTN, muscle wasting, osteoporosis, cushingoid appearance, ↓ wound healing, adrenal suppression, personality changes, fluid retention NSAIDs: dizziness, drowsiness, nausea, constipation, rashes, palpitations, ↑ bleeding time DMARDs: anemia, leukopenia, anorexia, nausea, chills, fever, rash, retinopathy, Raynaud phenomena **Contraind:** Hypersensitivity; NO NSAIDs if allergic to aspirin Steroids: NOT w/active untreated infections. **Use cautiously:** W/Hx of GI bleeding, diabetics DMARDs: NOT used in active infections, underlying malignancy, & uncontrolled diabetes

Antiulcer/Antacid

Antacids Aluminum hydroxide Magaldrate **Antiinfectives** Amoxicillin Clarithromycin **Histamine H$_2$-Receptor Antagonists** Cimetidine (Tagamet) Famotidine (Pepcid) Nizatidine (Axid) Ranitidine (Tritec) **Other** Esomeprazole (Nexium) Lansoprazole (Prevacid) Bismuth subsalicylate	**Indications:** Treat & prevent peptic ulcer or gastroesophageal reflux disease **Effect:** Antiinfective act on ***Helicobacter pylori,*** antacids neutralize stomach acid/protect ulcer surface from further damage **Common side effects:** May interfere w/ absorption of other oral meds, confusion, dizziness, drowsiness, ↓ sperm count, impotence, altered taste, black tongue **Contraind:** Hypersensitivity. **Use cautiously:** W/renal impairment & elderly

Antiviral

Acyclovir Amantadine Cidofovir Dososanol Famciclovir Foscarnet Ganciclovir Oseltamivir Penciclovir Ribavarin Valacyclovir Valganciclovir Vidarabine Zanamivir	**Indications:** Management of viruses: acyclovir: herpes virus & chickenpox; oseltamivir & zanamivir: influenza A; cidofovir, ganciclovir, valganciclovir, foscarnet: CMV; vidarabine: ophthalmic viruses **Effect:** Inhibit viral replication **Common side effects:** Acyclovir may cause CNS toxicity; foscarnet ↑ risk of seizures. **Other side effects:** Dizziness, HA, nausea, diarrhea, vomiting, trembling, pain, phlebitis, joint pain **Contrainds:** W/previous hypersensitivity. **Use cautiously:** W/renal impairment (dosage must be adjusted)

Bone Resorption Inhibitors

Alendronate (Fosamax) Etidronate (Didronel) Ibandronate (Boniva) Pamidronate (Aredia) Raloxifene (Evista)	**Indications:** Treatment & prevention of osteoporosis **Effect:** Inhibit bone resorption/inhibit osteoclast activity Bind to estrogen receptors

Continued

Risedronate (Actonel) Zoldronic acid (Reclast)	**Common side effects:** Abdominal pain, distention, constipation, diarrhea, musculoskeletal pain **Contraind:** Hypersensitivity, hypocalcemia, or women w/Hx of thromboembolic disease. **Use cautiously:** W/renal impairment
CNS Stimulants	
Amphetamine (Adderall) Dexmethylphenidate Dextroamphetamine Methylphenidate (Ritalin) Pemoline	**Indications:** Treatment of narcolepsy & management of ADHD **Effect:** ↑ levels of neurotransmitters in CNS, stimulation of respiratory & CNS, ↑ motor activity & mental alertness, ↓ sense of fatigue **Common side effects:** Hyperactivity, insomnia, tremor, HTN, palpitations, tachy, anorexia, constipation, dry mouth, rashes, hypersensitivity reactions **Contraind:** Hypersensitivity, pregnant & lactating women, hyperexcitable states. **Use cautiously:** W/psychotic personalities or suicidal/homicidal patient/clients w/Hx of CAD; diabetes; & elderly
Lipid Lowering	
Atorvastatin (Lipitor) Cholestyramine (Questran) Colesevelam (Welchol) Colestipol (Colestid) Rosuvastatin (Crestor) Fenofibrate (Tricor) Fluvastatin (Lescol) Gemfibrozil (Lopid) Lovastatin (Mevacor) Niacin (Niaspan) Pitavastatin (Livalo) Pravastatin (Pravachol) Simvastatin (Zocor) Vytorin Zetia	**Indications:** To ↓ blood lipids/↓ risk of morbidity & mortality of atherosclerotic CVD **Effect:** Inhibit enzymes in cholesterol synthesis or bind cholesterol in GI tract **Common side effects:** Abdominal discomfort, constipation, nausea, rashes Muscle pain/aching not associated w/ exercise; may be sign of toxicity to drug **Contraind:** Hypersensitivity, complete biliary obstruction. **Use cautiously:** W/Hx of constipation, liver disease

NSAIDs	
Aspirin Celecoxib (Celebrex) Choline salicylate Flurbiprofen Ibuprofen Indomethacin Ketoprofen Nabumetone Naproxen Oxaprozin Piroxicam Salsalate Sulindac Tolmetin Valdecoxib	**Indications:** Control of mild → mod pain, fever & inflammatory conditions: osteo- & rheumatoid arthritis **Effect:** Analgesia, anti-inflammatory, & ↓ fever; inhibits synthesis of prostaglandins **Common side effects:** Dizziness, drowsiness, nausea, constipation, palpitations, rashes, prolonged bleeding time **Contraind:** If allergic to aspirin: NO NSAIDs **Use cautiously:** W/Hx of bleeding disorders, including GI, & w/hepatic, renal & cardiovascular disease
Pain	
Acetaminophen Tramadol Hydrochloride (Ultracet) Acetaminophen codeine (Tylenol with codeine) Acetaminophen hydrocodone bitartrate (Vicodin or Lortab) Acetaminophen oxycodone hydrochloride (Percoset) Aspirin Butorphanol tartrate (Stadol) Demerol (Meperidine) Dilaudid (hydromorphone) Etodolac (Lodine) Hydrocodone bitartrate ibuprofen (Vicoprofen) Ketoprofen (Orudis) Naproxen (Naprosyn) Fentanyl citrate (Duragesic) Mefenamic acid Meperidine hydrochloride Buprenorphine (Buprenex) Levophanol tartrate (Levo-Dromoran)	**Indications:** Relieves pain from multitudes of causes **Common side effects:** Shallow breathing, slow heart beat, seizure (convulsions), cold clammy skin, sweating, confusion, severe weakness, dizziness or feeling like might pass out, nausea, vomiting, constipation, loss of appetite, HA, tired feeling, dry mouth, itching **Use cautiously:** Can be habit forming Impairs judgment & should not be used when making important decisions or operating vehicles

Continued

Morphine sulfate
Nalburphine hydrochloride
(Nubain)
OxyContin (oxycodone
hydrochloride)
Toradol
Tramadol hydrochloride

Peripheral Arterial Hypertension

Adcirca (tadalafil) Flolan (epoprostenol) Isordil Letairis (ambrisentan) Remodulin (treprosinil) Revatio (sildenafil) Tracleer (bosentan) Tyvaso (treprostinil) Veletri Ventavis (iloprostenol)	**Indications:** Vasodilators: relax smooth muscle to increase blood flow to certain areas of body, particularly peripheral arterial vasodilation **Common side effects:** Hypotension, dizziness or feeling light-headed, fainting, vision changes

Sedatives

Ambien (zolpidem) Atarax (hydroxyzine) Ativan (lorazepam) Luminol (phenobarbital) Lunesta (eszopiclone) Nembutol (pentobarbital) Phenergan (promethazine) Seconal (secobarbitol) Vistaril (hydroxyzine)	**Indications:** Treat insomnia, or decrease anxiety (Ativan); can slow activity of brain and/or nervous system. Can be used pre-surgery to relax individuals **Common side effects:** Chest pain, fast or irregular heart beat, feeling short of breath, trouble breathing or swallowing, aggressive behavior, hallucinations, daytime drowsiness, dizziness, or feeling like might pass out, weakness, feeling "drugged" or light-headed, fatigue, loss of coordination, dry mouth, nose or throat irritation, nausea, constipation, diarrhea, upset stomach, stuffy nose, sore throat, HA, muscle pain

Skeletal Muscle Relaxants

Baclofen Carisoprodol Chlorzoxazone Cyclobenzaprine Dantrolene Diazepam Metaxalone Methocarbamol Orphenadrine	**Indications:** Management of spasticity in spinal cord injury & relief of pain in acute musculoskeletal conditions **Effect:** Centrally acting (all except dantrolene) Inhibits reflexes at spinal level & may affect bowel & bladder function **Common side effects:** Nausea, dizziness, drowsiness, fatigue, weakness, constipation, hyperglycemia. May cause muscle weakness. **Contraind:** In patient/clients who use spasticity for functional activities including posture & balance. **Use cautiously:** W/previous liver disease

Medical Wellness Screening

Type	Tests Recommended	Recommendations
Breast Cancer Screening	Self-Exam Clinical Breast Exam	Monthly Every 2–3 y, age 20–39 Annually for women >39
	Mammogram	Annually @ age >39 Women w/previous Hx of breast CA, documented genetic mutation &/or strong family Hx of breast CA should have mammogram earlier than 40 w/ultrasound &/or MRI
	Genetic Testing	*If* strong family Hx of breast or ovarian CA
Cardiovascular Disease Screening	PAR-Q Cholesterol Triglycerides HDL LDL HDL/Cholesterol Risk Ratio Blood Pressure Check Stress Test C-Reactive Protein Berkeley Lab Test	Par-Q before starting an exercise program Lab work for those w/family Hx C-reactive protein & Berkeley Lab Tests for those w/family Hx of heart disease Stress testing for those w/ Sx or moderate to high risk of developing disease
Colon Cancer Screening	Colonoscopy	Regular screening @ age 50 (unless family Hx) Colonoscopy at 50 & every 10 y
	Flexible Sigmoidoscopy High-Sensitivity Decal Occult Blood Test	Every 5 y after 50 Every y after 50

Medical Wellness Screening—cont'd		
Type	**Tests Recommended**	**Recommendations**
Diabetes Screening	Blood Glucose HbA1c	Screen for type 2 diabetes in adults w/BP >135/80
Gastrointestinal Disorders	Total & Direct Bilirubin Alkaline Phosphatase Serum Glutamic Oxaloacetic Transaminase (SGOT) Serum Glutamic Pyruvic Transaminase (SGPT) Gamma-Glutamyl Transpeptidase (GGT) Lactate Dehydrogenase (LDH) Albumin Total Protein	Screen only if individuals present w/strong family Hx or Sx
Therapeutic Exercise Screening	Cardiovascular Disease Screening Musculoskeletal Dysfunction Neuromuscular/Balance Dysfunction	PAR Q & You & Risk Factor Profile Musculoskeletal quick screen Balance quick screen
Kidney Function Screening	Blood Urea Nitrogen (BUN) Creatinine Estimated Glomerular Filtration Rate (eGFR) Phosphorus Sodium Potassium Chloride Calcium Uric Acid Magnesium	Screen only if individuals present w/strong family Hx, Sx, or other diseases that can affect kidney functioning
Ovarian Cancer Screening	Serum Ca-125 Transvaginal Ultrasound	For women w/increased or inherited risk

Continued

Medical Wellness Screening—cont'd

Type	Tests Recommended	Recommendations
Peripheral Arterial Disease Screening	Ankle Brachial Index Test Risk Factor Profile for CAD	Screen in individuals w/ other cardiovascular disease & those w/Sx
Prostate Cancer Screening	Digital Rectal Exam	Yearly for men >49
	Prostate Specific Antigen (PSA)	Annual PSA for men >49; possibly early if family Hx
Skin Cancer screening	Whole body mole check by dermatologist	Yearly exam
Thyroid Screening	Thyroxine (T4)	Insufficient evidence to regularly screen Screen if Sx indicate potential problem

Physical Activity Readiness Questionnaire for People Ages 15–69 (PARQ)

1. __ Yes __ No   Has your doctor ever said that you have a heart condition and that you should only do physical activity recommended by a doctor?
2. __ Yes __ No   Do you feel pain in your chest when you do physical activity?
3. __ Yes __ No   In the past month, have you had chest pain when you were not doing physical activity?
4. __ Yes __ No   Do you lose your balance because of dizziness or do you ever lose consciousness?
5. __ Yes __ No   Do you have a bone or joint problem (for example, back, knee, or hip) that could be made worse by a change in your physical activity?

6. __ Yes __ No   Are you currently taking medication (e.g., water pills) for your blood pressure or heart condition?
7. __ Yes __ No   Do you know of any other reason why you should not do physical activity?

If you answered *yes* to *any* question above:

- Talk with your doctor by phone or in person *before* you start becoming much more physically active or *before* you have a fitness appraisal. Tell your doctor about the PAR-Q and which questions you answered *yes*.
- You may be able to do any activity you want—as long as you start slowly and build up gradually. Or, you may need to restrict your activities to those that are safe for you. Talk with your doctor about the activities you wish to participate in and follow his or her advice.
- Find out which community programs are safe and helpful for you.

If you answered *no* to *all* questions above:*

- Start becoming much more physically active—begin slowly and build up gradually. This is the safest and easiest way to go.
- Take part in a fitness appraisal—this is an excellent way to determine your basic fitness so you can plan the best way for you to live actively. It is also highly recommended that you have your blood pressure evaluated. If your reading is over 144/94, talk with your doctor before you start becoming much more physically active.

* Delay starting exercise program if you are feeling ill, or if you are or may be pregnant.
Printed with permission Canadian Society for Exercise Physiology, www.csep.ca. Arraix et al, 1992. Reading, 1992.

Exercise Recommendations for Lower Back & Core Region

An individualized program is the best; everyone has different flexibility, strength, and alignment. The following, however, are recommended beginner's exercises to prevent back injury.

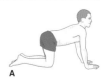

A

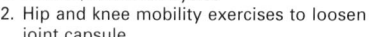

2. Hip and knee mobility exercises to loosen joint capsule
3. Strengthening of anterior abdominal muscles w/spine in neutral
4. Strengthening of lateral muscles of side support for quadratus lumborum & abdominal wall
5. Strengthening of extensor muscles
6. Stabilization exercises including posterior pelvic tilt

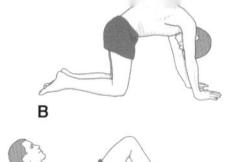

Screening for abdominal endurance: Patient/client performs 25 partial curl-ups within 1 min

Screening for upper body strength: Push-ups performed in 1 min

Things to Consider With Exercise Program for the Back

■ These exercises should be performed daily
■ There should *not* be any pain when doing these exercises
■ Strengthening exercises, aerobic, & cardiovascular exercises should also be included
■ It is *not* recommended to do these exercises upon first rising out of bed in AM due to potential lack of fluid/ lubrication of vertebral discs

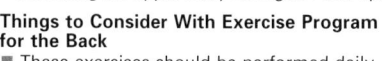

(McGill, 1998.)

Risk Stratification for Heart Disease			
	Low Risk	**Moderate Risk**	**High Risk**
Risk factors for heart disease	Asymptomatic ≤1 total risk factor	≥2 total risk factors	Symptomatic, or known cardiac, pulmonary, or metabolic disease

Risk Stratification—cont'd			
	Low Risk	**Moderate Risk**	**High Risk**
Medical exam and GXT before exercise?	Moderate exercise: not necessary Vigorous exercise: not necessary	Moderate exercise: not necessary Vigorous exercise: recommended	Moderate exercise: recommended Vigorous exercise: recommended
Doctor supervision of exercise test?	Submaximal: not necessary Maximal: not necessary	Submaximal: not necessary Maximal: recommended	Submaximal: recommended Maximal: recommended

Adapted from ACSM Guidelines for exercise testing and prescription, ed. 7. Lippincott Williams & Wilkins, Philadelphia, 2006.

RISK FACTOR ANALYSES FOR HEART DISEASE AND PULMONARY DYSFUNCTION: SEE CARDIO TAB

Emerging Risk Factors: CAD/Atherosclerosis

- Homocysteine
- C-reactive protein
- Lp(a)
- Thrombolytic factors (look at PT/PTT values)
- Endothelial dysfunction (↑ reactivity of arteries/arterioles: vasospasm or ↑ release of EDRF, resulting in ↑ LDL adhesion & atherosclerosis)
- Obesity
- Elevated triglycerides
- Hyperinsulinemia
- Glucose intolerance
- Decreased HDLs
- Metabolic syndrome: three or more of the following
  - Insulin resistance
  - Abnormal uric acid metabolism
  - Increased plasma uric acid concentration
  - ↓ renal clearance of uric acid

COPD Population Screener

1. During the past 4 weeks, how much of the time did you feel short of breath?
( ) none of the time (0)
( ) a little of the time (0)
( ) some of the time (1)
( ) most of the time (2)
( ) all of the time (2)

2. Do you ever cough up any "stuff," such as mucus or phlegm?
( ) no, never (0)
( ) only with occasional colds or chest infections (0)
( ) yes, a few days a month (1)
( ) yes, most days a week (1)
( ) yes, every day (2)

3. Please select the answer that best describes you in the past 12 months. I do less than I used to because of my breathing problems.
( ) strongly disagree (0)
( ) disagree (0)
( ) unsure (0)
( ) agree (1)
( ) strongly agree (2)

4. Have you smoked at least 100 cigarettes in your *entire* life?
( ) no (0)
( ) yes (2)
( ) don't know (0)

5. How old are you?
( ) age 35–49 (0)
( ) age 50–59 (1)
( ) age 60–69 (2)
( ) age 70+ (2)

Score Screener by adding points from questions 1 through 5.
Total Score = _____
If total score is ≥5, this means your breathing problems may be caused by chronic obstructive pulmonary disease (COPD).
0–4 = LOW risk of COPD

Epworth Sleepiness Scale*

How likely are you to doze off or fall asleep in the following situations, in contrast to feeling just tired?

Use the most appropriate number from the following scale for each situation. Answer all questions to your best ability. 0 = would never doze 2 = moderate chance 1 = slight chance of dozing 3 = high chance of dozing	
SITUATION	**Chance of Dozing (0–3)**
Sitting and reading	
Watching TV	
Sitting inactive in a public place (e.g., a theatre or a meeting)	
As a passenger in a car for an hour without a break	
Lying down to rest in the afternoon when circumstances permit	
Sitting and talking to someone	
Sitting quietly after a lunch without alcohol	
In a car while stopped for a few minutes in traffic	
TOTAL SCORE	
Score: 0–24, the higher the number, the greater the sleepiness. Normal Range: 0–10	

*Reproduced with permission Dr. Murray Johns mjohns@optalert.com

Equations for Prediction of Basal Metabolic Rate Based on Wt

	Males		Females
Age (y)	**kcal/d**	**Age (y)**	**Kcal/D**
18–30	15.3 × wt in kg + 679	18–31	14.7 × wt in kg + 496
30–60	11.6 × wt in kg + 879	30–61	8.7 × wt in kg + 829
>60	13.5 × wt in kg + 487	>61	10.5 × wt in kg + 596

Primary Components of Healthy Wt Loss Program

Total Calories	Women: no fewer than 1200 cal/d Men: no fewer than 1500 cal/d
Fat	<30% cal, ↓ sat fat & *trans*-fatty acids
Protein	20%–25% cal, no fewer than 75 g/d
Carbohydrates	50% of cal, not <5 servings of fruits & vegetables ↓ simple sugars, ↑complex sugars (starches)
Dietary fiber	20–30 g/d from food sources
Water	Not less than 1 L/d
Alcohol	Limit intake

Interventions for Optimal Wellness

Intervention	Potential Outcomes
Vaccines	Prevention of disease
Diet	↓ risk of obesity & obesity-related diseases such as diabetes, cardiovascular disease, etc
Exercise	Maintenance of normal body wt, aerobic capacity, flexibility, & ↓ risk of disease

Interventions for Optimal Wellness—cont'd

Intervention	Potential Outcomes
Sunblock	Prevention of burn injury Prevention of skin CA
Seatbelt use	Prevention of head or other serious injury/or death in a car accident
Ergonomic adjustment for worksite	Prevention of work-related injuries such as CTS, back, neck
Risk factor assessment including family Hx	Prevention of disease or early detection of disease before potential harm or dysfunction
Medical wellness screenings at recommended ages	Prevention of disease
Skin checks	Prevention or early detection of skin CA
Helmet use	Prevention of concussion: use with high-risk head injury like certain sports, motorcycles, etc.

Guide to PT Practice Patterns for Wellness

Pattern Number	Description
4A	Primary Prevention/Risk Reduction for Skeletal Demineralization
5A	Primary Prevention/Risk Reduction for Loss of Balance and Falling
6A	Primary Prevention/Risk Reduction for Cardiovascular/Pulmonary Disorders
7A	Primary Prevention/Risk Reduction for Integumentary Disorders

REFERENCES

Agency for Healthcare Research and Quality, Classification Guidelines, Rockville, MD, http://www.ahrq.gov/2012

American Medical Association. Current Procedural Terminology, http://ama-assn.org/ama/pub/physician-resources/solutions-managing-your-practice/coding-billing-insurance/cpt.page?, 2011.

American Physical Therapy Association. Defensible Documentation for Patient/Client Management. Alexandria, VA, http://apta.org/Documentation/Defensible Documentation/ 2012

American Physical Therapy Association. Guide to Physical Therapist Practice, ed. 2. Phys Ther 2001;81:9–744.

Arraix GA, Wigle DT, Mao Y. Risk assessment of physical activity and physical fitness in the Canada Health Survey Follow-Up Study. J. Clin. Epidemiol 1992;45:419–428.

Calisir C, Yavas US, Ozkan IR, et al. Performance of the Wells and revised Geneva scores for predicting pulmonary embolism. Eur J Emerg Med 2009;16:49–52.

Centers for Medicare and Mediacid Services. Medicare Coverage Database. cms.hs.gov/mcd/search.asp;aacvpr.org

Dole RL, Chafetz R. Pediatrics Rehabilitation Notes. Philadelphia: FA Davis, 2010.

Filipek et al. The screening and diagnosis of autistic spectrum disorders. J Autism Develop Disorder 1999 Dec;29(6):439–84.

Greenspan S, I, & Wieder, S. A functional developmental approach to autism spectrum disorders. Journal of the Association for Persons with Severe Handicaps (JASH), 1999;24 (3): 147–161

Guccione, A. Geriatric Physical Therapy, ed. 3. Elsevier-Mosby; St. Louis, 2012.

Gulick D. Ortho Notes, ed. 2. F.A. Davis: Philadelphia; 2009, p. 133.

Hartman K. Outcomes of routine episiotomy. JAMA 2005;293:2141.

Klok FA, Kruisman E, Spaan J, et al. Comparison of the revised Geneva score with the Wells rule for assessing clinical probability of pulmonary embolism. J Thromb Haemost 2008;6:40–44.

Le Gal G, Righini M, Roy RM, et al. Prediction of pulmonary embolism in the emergency department: The revised Geneva score. Ann Intern Med 2006;144:165–171.

McGill SM. Low back exercises: Evidence for improving exercise regimens. *Phys Ther* 1998;78;7:754.

Ozer M, Payton O, Nelson C. *Treatment Planning for Rehabilitation: A Patient-Centered Approach.* McGraw-Hill, New York, 2000, pp. 37, 60.

Ozonoff S. (2003). Early identification of autism. M.I.N.D. Summer Institute on Neurodevelopmental Disorders, Sacramento, CA.

Thomas S, Reading J, Shephard RJ. Revision of the Physical Activity Readiness Questionnaire (PAR-Q). *Can J Sport Sci* 1992;17:4 338–345.

World Health Organization. International Statistical Classification of Diseases, ed. 10. Geneva: 2010. http://apps.who.int/classifications/icd10/browse/2010/en

INDEX